Womb Medicine

The Art of Yoni Steaming for Women's Health

Sali McIntyre

FOREWORD BY DR. ROSITA ARVIGO

adpublishing

A self-published title
Animal Dreaming Publishing
www.AnimalDreamingPublishing.com

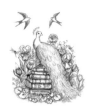

Womb Medicine
A self-published book produced with the help and support of

ANIMAL DREAMING PUBLISHING
PO Box 5203 East Lismore NSW 2480
AUSTRALIA
Phone +61 2 6622 6147
www.AnimalDreamingPublishing.com
www.facebook.com/AnimalDreamingPublishing

First published in 2020

Copyright text © Sali McIntyre
www.heartandsoulofwellness.com.au
www.facebook.com/heartandsoulofwellnesscentre

Cover image © Melissa Juchau
www.facebook.com/Melissaonebeing

Internal images © Kamimi Art, Melissa Juchau, Olga Korneeva,
Fandorina Liza, Andy Permana Putra

ISBN 978-0-6486508-8-1

Disclaimer All information in this book is offered for educational purposes
only. Please consider and consult professionals in the relevant field to
make an educated decision as to whether suggestions in this book are
right for you.

Printed in China

Author's Note

Each year many women are diagnosed with cervical cancer, fibroids, cysts, Polycystic Ovary Syndrome (PCOS) and other gynaecological issues. Surgery is lifesaving when it is needed. However, many women are accepting surgery as the first option to deal with their symptoms rather than investigating less invasive procedures first. Yoni steaming is a non-invasive, nourishing ritual women can comfortably practise at home to nurture their womb health and deepen their own body intuition to know what is best for them.

To all my loved ones.
This book is about the beauty of women's wisdom.
May we all benefit from its re-emergence.

I acknowledge the Bundjalung tribe, the traditional
custodians of the land – where I live in the beautiful
cauldron of Mt Warning – and the Elders past,
present and future.

I honour my own Anglo-Celtic ancestry and
the traditional healing practices of indigenous
cultures the world over.

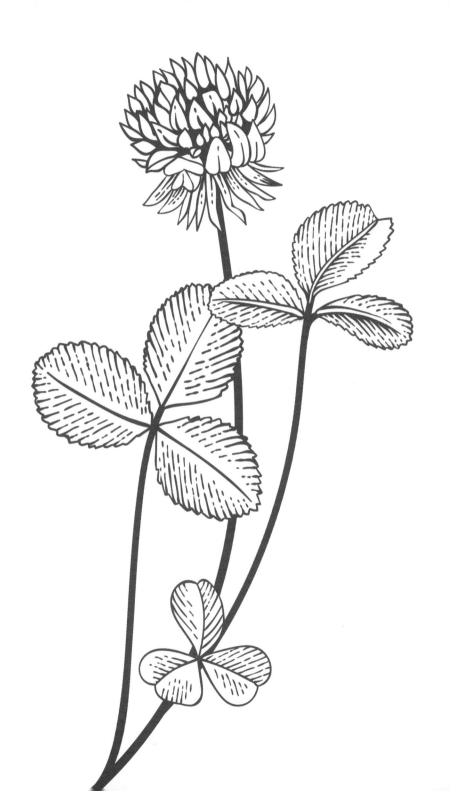

Contents

Foreword

Sali McIntyre is a midwife, birth keeper and Arvigo®
practitioner. Her passion for women's reproductive health,
pregnancy wellness and postpartum health makes her
just the right person to pen this book on yoni steams. I first
met Sali four years ago when she attended a workshop
I conducted in Belize on The Arvigo Techniques of Maya
Abdominal Therapy®. Through these techniques and her
own extensive background in women's health, Sali has
assisted countless women to achieve better reproductive
health. Her much-awaited book on yoni steaming
describes and explains this technique practiced all over
the world since ancient times. In my travels, I have met
women and healers from Central and South America,
Egypt, Turkey, Greece and Italy who are familiar with
this practice, though, sadly many do not practice it
any longer. Native American women told me that they
remember grandmothers and aunties who gave yoni
steams to women of all ages. Mennonite women of
German descent remember the practice but now few
remember how to do them. In Mexico, Guatemala and

Belize Maya healers still recommend yoni steams for women's health. In my Naprapathic practice in Belize, one of my Mennonite patients, brought me an old home remedy book published in 1910 with a drawing of a woman taking a yoni steam. Sali's well written, heartfelt book will go a long way to re-introduce this vital healing modality to women and girls all over the globe.

I first learned of the practice in 1985 from my own mentors, Hortence Robinson, a herbal midwife in Belize and Elijio Panti, a shaman-healer also of Belize, both now deceased. Hortence and Elijio relied on external abdominal/pelvic massage, herbal remedies and yoni steams for women's health. When women came to Hortence or Elijio with menstrual or reproductive complaints, the first question they inevitably asked was "Well, did you do a vaginal steam?" That is a question I heard many elders ask women again and again over the years. As a doctor of Naprapathy for the past forty years, my own practice in the United States and Belize was focused on women and children, thus it was a natural progression for me to include the massage techniques and yoni steams I learned from my indigenous mentors. I first introduced yoni steams into my classes in Arvigo Techniques of Maya Abdominal Therapy® as early as 1990. Since then the practice has undergone a much-deserved renaissance in the field of women's health and self-care modalities.

Maya people have long known about yoni steams to relieve menstrual pains, uterine pathologies and always for post-partum care. In Yucatan, Mexico on the island of Cozumel the early Spanish friars wrote of an ancient temple site dedicated to Ix Chel, the Maya Goddess of Fertility and Healing. Here, women from all over the Known World made two pilgrimages in a lifetime to the holy site to seek healing and fertility. The first journey they made was in menarche when young women, recently made fertile through the onset of menstruation went to worship the Goddess and to pray for fertility and successful birth outcomes. In menopause, after fertility waned, women made the pilgrimage again in thanksgiving for their children. Here at the ancient temple, women pilgrims received the abdominal/pelvic massage, yoni steams, full body steam baths, herbal teas and time to rest, meditate and enjoy the cooling ocean breezes. Women and girls came on foot over causeways paved with white marl earth or in canoes from coastal areas near and far. To insure that the island would be accessible to all pilgrims, they were housed at state-supported inns along the pilgrim's way. Cozumel Island was a women's sanctuary for healing and a place to study astronomy, calendrics, weaving, midwifery and the art of divination. Victims of domestic violence were welcomed, protected and healed of their emotional and physical traumas. They could, if they wished, spend the rest of their lives in safety with other women and children. Orphans were brought there to be raised by infertile women who were often rejected by their husbands and families. How we need such a sanctuary now. Wouldn't it be grand?

Exactly what does a yoni steam do? Sali offers her reader a full explanation and description of the practice whose basic ingredients are water, plants and steam. Sali explains that some, like myself, include prayer. In times of dire need like hurricanes, fires, drought or even famine, women have used only water and salt to great effect. Miss Hortence told me the story of birthing her seventh child during a raging Category 5 hurricane in Belize. She and her children lived in a two-room wooden house alongside a creek. Her other children were sent to stay with their grandmother down the road while, unattended, Hortence lay on her bed giving birth. The baby was born as the creek water rose to two feet within the house. When this happens, there is always debris from out houses floating in the rising waters. Hortence wrapped her baby and its placenta in a towel and braved the raging storm to get to her mother's in knee deep filthy water. Her mother, also a midwife, immediately cut the umbilical cord, bathed the baby, wrapped it up then gave Hortence a yoni steam with only water and salt. She said that after the steam she passed the largest post-partum clots she had ever seen in twenty years of midwifery.

This book will teach you what you need to know about yoni steams to do them at home or in a professional setting. As Sali explains, there are many plants suitable for yoni steams, yet every practitioner has their favourites. Mine are mugwort, basil, oregano, rosemary, thyme, roses and hibiscus. In Belize, I have a sixteen-acre farm in the middle of a verdant rainforest reserve, so I am able to grow these plants year-round in my tropical garden. You will learn in these pages which plants can be used, how to prepare them for yoni steams, what contraindications to consider and what to expect after steams.

I am thrilled to introduce this important book to Sali's readers and I know it will become a classic in the field of women's health.

Dr Rosita Arvigo, DN
Author, lecturer and Founder of The Arvigo Techniques of Maya Abdominal Therapy®
Ix Chel Tropical Research Centre
San Ignacio, Belize, Central America

Introduction

WOMB HEALING MEDICINE: ANCIENT WOMEN'S WISDOM

I see a startled or intrigued expression on many women's faces the first time I mention yoni (vaginal) steaming. I have found that the look of incredulity is quickly followed by curiosity, a desire to know more before asking, 'How can I get one of those?' I resonate deeply with these women as it wasn't too long ago that I had the same expression and feelings. Prior to coming across the Arvigo Techniques of Maya Abdominal Therapy®, I had never heard of vaginal steaming. I'd never heard of womb massage either, for that matter.

I have long been interested in women's health, being a woman, mother, yoga teacher and midwife. Since I own hundreds of textbooks and books on women's health, it puzzled me that I had never heard of such practices.

Medicine women healers and shamans of many cultures have forever used their knowledge of herbs to help women heal their bodies. Before modern medicine there was no other way. Women's lore was handed down from mother to daughter and from medicine woman to apprentice.

At some point in history, the widespread teachings of this practice ceased. History tells us that the Spaniards burned the books of traditional Mayan medicine techniques. Perhaps this is why this powerful medicine is not well known today. For many generations we have been governed by a patriarchal society whereby women's traditional medicine and knowledge have been discounted as superstitious 'old wives' tales. With the rise of feminine consciousness, it is becoming more apparent that these 'old wives' were wise women and that their tales offer proven options for modern day problems.

Now these old ways are being revealed to the Western world for greater holistic healing. We can surmise that grassroot medicine such as yoni steaming does not make money for big corporations. However, the collective is open to its re-emergence and women are embracing this practice with open arms and open hearts.

Yoni steaming received prominent attention in the media three years ago when Gwyneth Paltrow espoused the benefits of the 'V-Steam' on her lifestyle blog. She claimed it was an energetic release and that it helped balance female hormones. This caused an outcry among medical doctors who countered that there was no scientific evidence supporting its merits.

It is true that the benefit of vaginal steaming does not have the backup of scientific or medical research. By the same token, there is no scientific research to say it doesn't work. Anecdotal evidence is growing like wildflowers and I know that this treatment will eventually gain mainstream recognition as women discover its healing benefits and medical doctors observe its potent effects.

Yoni Steaming for Modern Times

Yoni steaming has been practised by almost every indigenous culture in the world.

The sacred knowledge of *bajos* (steam bath) and *la saboda* (womb massage) has been passed down from the ancient lineage of Maya medicine from Don Elijio Panti, Miss Hortense Robinson and other traditional herbal midwives in Central America to Rosita Arvigo. For the most part, vaginal steaming was unknown in the Western world until Rosita brought the wisdom and teachings of Maya healing and womb massage to America and later, other countries.

As this work grows and flourishes in the West, so it has found its way to Australia. At present, Australia has fifty Arvigo® practitioners, and the teachings and practice of yoni steaming is becoming more well known.

My Story

I am not a herbalist nor a Traditional Chinese Medicine practitioner. I do not claim to have the knowledge or expertise to cure chronic ailments. Apart from my own research and the online tutorials I have done with Steamy Chick (see Resources), I have no formal training in this area. This knowledge is being passed down once again from woman to woman. The information I present comes from the Arvigo® lineage of Maya healing, within which I practice, and from what my colleagues and myself have discovered through our own work with our clients. Since this book's inception I have learnt so much about vaginal steaming and am still learning about vaginal steam protocols for different reproductive conditions based on a woman's menstrual history.

I am curious about which herbs women are using for yoni steams and I admire their willingness and courage to try new combinations. Personally, I would never have thought to use cinnamon, turmeric or sea moss. Roots, bark and berries are also being tried in the steams. As herbalists and practitioners keep records of our restorative plant allies and their healing effects, knowledge of the most appropriate herbs will grow.

Since this book had its beginnings two years ago, there is now an exponential wealth of information about the practice of yoni steaming on the worldwide web. There are many, many yoni steam blends and products on the internet market that can be sent to you from all around the world. I still think it is wise to get to know and love the plants in your own garden in your own corner of the world. Do your own trials. Ask for guidance. Trust your intuition. We hear that a lot I know, but also trust your common sense.

I have dried herbs picked from my garden hung in bunches everywhere in my kitchen. I let the herbs guide my intuition. As my knowledge of which herbs are suitable for which ailments grow, I will refine this practice. The old adage comes to mind: *First Do No Harm*.

Keep in mind that some herbs may cause allergic reactions. If your steam session causes vulva irritation or itchiness, please discontinue immediately.

The herbal blends I recommend are generic ones that will have a gentle cleansing effect on the uterus. The herbs I have listed are ones that I am familiar with and for the most part these herbs grow in Northern New South Wales, Australia, where I live.

This book is designed to stimulate your interest in this topic. Hopefully I have shone the light on herbs, their magical properties and their willingness to bring beauty and healing into your life. It is not intended to be taken as gospel particularly when it comes to choosing herbs to cure a certain ailment or imbalance.

I believe yoni steaming will be a beautiful addition to your women's medicine bag and that it should rightfully take its place there. Choosing a healthy non-toxic diet and lifestyle, a healing mindset, and the guidance of a qualified herbalist and/or natural health practitioner are recommended.

∽

Uterine steaming unites the female body with the plant medicine world, using nature as it was intended, to heal dis-ease. It gives us women the opportunity to celebrate, cherish and love our bodies, and enjoy our wombs and vaginas for the beautiful sacred gifts they are.

—Tracey Whitton

∽

Discovering the Arvigo® Techniques has had a profound influence on my life. Seeking out a practitioner even a few years ago was not easy. My first session was with Danielle Rickwood, in Byron Bay. When she talked about her womb as a 'she' I had one of those 'ah ha' moments. If every woman talked about her womb as a she as if she was someone you could connect with and receive guidance from then I believe our world would shift on its axis.

Having had a radical hysterectomy at the age of thirty-four, there was a part of me that felt I had missed out on the renaissance of connecting with my womb as my best friend and celebrating my menstrual cycle as a spiritual messenger. No matter how many people told me that the energetic blueprint of my womb still remained, I never quite believed it.

Feelings of low self-worth and body shame led to many years of looking everywhere outside of myself for validation. Dropping out of my head and into my heart space and further into my womb space, I have become aware that the journey towards unconditional self-love is a long and winding yet necessary path to travel. Furthermore, no amount of external recognition, courses, workshops and/or new projects will complete the journey. This is an inward process. Choosing to listen to the voice of compassion and self-love instead of the inner critic will always be a daily practice for me.

୨ଝ

When you befriend your female body and her inherent wisdom, you are more likely to be kinder to yourself and make lifestyle choices that enhance health and wellbeing and feelings of self-love and acknowledgment.

୨ଝ

My initiation into vaginal steaming took place at an Arvigo® Self-Care weekend in inner-city Melbourne with Andrea Lopez—one of the very first healers to bring this work to Australia. For many years, Andrea was the creatrix behind the Womb Room—a mobile womb tent that she set up at markets introducing and educating women about yoni steaming and womb wisdom.

From there, I found myself on a trajectory that took me across the world to train with the Arvigo Institute and take every course on offer, including Advanced Pregnancy. Along the way I have met my Arvigo® tribe from whom I continue to receive an abundance of love support and mentorship. I am now a Certified Arvigo® Practitioner and Arvigo® Self-Care Instructor. I had the privilege of studying Spiritual Healing with Rosita Arvigo in Belize in 2016. The gratitude I feel is infinitely overflowing.

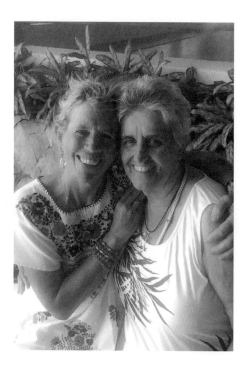

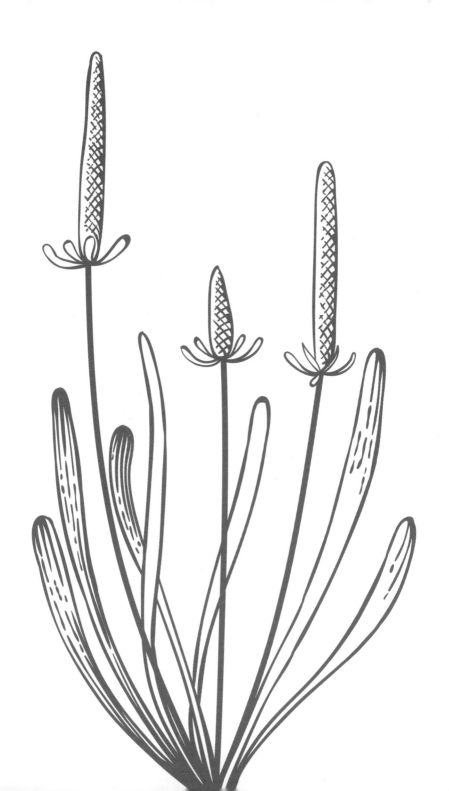

Chapter 1

What is a Yoni Steam?

Now known by many names, such as vaginal steaming, V-steaming, pelvic floor steaming and peri-steam hydrotherapy, a yoni steam is a simple practice that entails sitting or squatting over a pot of steaming herbs. I like to use the term 'yoni steam'. 'Yoni' is the Sanskrit word meaning 'sacred temple' or 'divine space' and refers to the entire female reproductive system including the exterior vulva, the vagina and the internal womb. All these parts benefit from the medicinal properties of the yoni steaming herbs.

Yoni steaming is accessible, affordable and you can do it at home. For further details refer to *Chapter 7: The Ingredients of a Yoni Steam* and *Chapter 8: How to do a Yoni Steam at Home.*

꧁꧂

*A yoni steam empowers women to have autonomy
over their own gynaecological wellbeing and treats
just about every problem known to gynaecology. It's also
a very effective prevention tool. It's the ultimate survival
guide to being a woman.*

—Keli Gaza

꧁꧂

Women are seeking more gentle and non-invasive ways of healing and are sharing this knowledge with each other as they take back responsibility for their own health.

A yoni steam is not a form of douching. The steam is not super-heated or forced into the uterus. Yoni steams bring healing warmth to the womb and to the pelvic floor increasing circulation and energy flow to the pelvis. This simple practice restores moisture, vitality and integrity to the vaginal tissues that are very porous and absorbent.

From a Mystical Perspective

More and more women are waking up and realising that they are disconnected from their womb centre. Within our womb centres we have a physical womb as well as a metaphysical womb. Yoni steaming cleanses the physical womb (if present) as well as the metaphysical womb. Our metaphysical womb is our connection with divine higher consciousness: our inner wisdom.

Many women—and you may be one of them— have never paid much attention to their womb and therefore feel cut off from this part of themselves. Do you live in your head and have forgotten how to tune in and trust your intuition about what is best for you? Do you take your body for granted and place an unrealistic expectation on it to perform on demand? In a fast-paced world, women are not encouraged to take the time to slow down and rest as their natural energy cycle waxes and wanes with the moon and the tides, especially during menstruation. Plant medicine has been replaced with the convenience of analgesics that mask the symptoms. However, analgesics do not address the underlying causes of pain discomfort and illness like traditional plant medicine does. A yoni steam practice provides space for women to connect with the divinity of their being and to align with the healing powers of the universe to naturally treat ailments on all levels.

FROM AN ENERGETIC PERSPECTIVE

Energy medicine is complementary to mainstream medicine and can be a complete self-care system in itself. It is based on the premise that all things, including the trillions of cells that make up your physical body, radiate energy. Utilising techniques from ancient healing modalities such as acupuncture, qigong and kinesiology, energy flow is enhanced and the body bought back to balance. Reiki, tapping, flower essences and crystal healing work on the same principles. As we explore these therapeutic paths for healing and wellbeing we are given more options to address our health concerns in a safe, gentle and time-honoured way.

Most people (and you might be an exception) don't 'see' their energy body with their physical eyes. Nor do you 'see' the energy centres that are lined up along your spine. These spinning wheels of energy (as described by people who do see them) are known as chakras and correspond to the major endocrine glands of your body. They interrelate with your physical body sending and receiving information from the external world like radio transmitters. Each chakra reflects the health of a particular area of the body. Blocked energy in any of your chakras can lead to illness.

The sacral chakra is the chakra associated with the reproductive organs and sexuality. It is where creativity happens. Think of your sacral chakra as an energetic gateway; a door to your intuition. When this chakra is balanced, one is physically healthy, grounded, intuitive and able to maintain healthy emotional boundaries. When out of balance there may be menstrual irregularities, issues with the lower back, sacrum and hips, or lack of self-esteem and concerns about body image. Anger, anxiety, shame and trauma can all manifest as disease in this part of your body.

\)๑ฺ(

The gift of yoni steaming goes way,
way beyond its physical benefits.

\)๑ฺ(

Your womb is your birthing centre for creation whether you wish to grow a child, a business or any creative endeavour. Creating a practice to nurture this creative temple where all things grow is so vital in these times of stress. Stress is the cause of many illnesses and women men and children alike suffer from anxiety and depression.

Yoni steaming brings energy healing into your life. The feeling of energy rising and healing is undeniable and is especially potent when combined with the loving restorative power of Mother Nature and her plant allies.

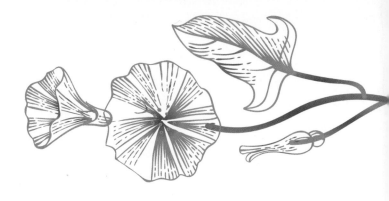

Yoni steaming is a sacred meditation and will reconnect you to your feminine body and the wisdom of plant medicine.

The practice is a powerfully fulfilling experience that rejuvenates body mind and soul. As it relaxes the nervous system, yoni steaming offers the potential for you to go deep within to awaken and fire up energy residing at the base of your spine. In yogic philosophy this is known as 'the awakening of kundalini energy'. Clearing blockages in the lower chakras enables kundalini energy to rise, enhancing connection with self. The sacred steaming ritual is also a wonderful way to practice meditation and mindfulness.

Yoni steaming with herbs offers an opportunity to deepen your spiritual practice: cleanse away the old and make space for the new.

Yoni mudra

In yogic philosophy, a mudra is a hand gesture that channels your body's energy flow.

A yoni mudra symbolises the vulva and will assist you to tune inwards and detach from the outer world. By making this downward pointing triangle shape with your hands, you access shakti, your inner feminine power. Practicing this mudra while you sit and steam will aid feelings of centredness and grounding. Adding mindfulness and breath awareness will further enrich your experience.

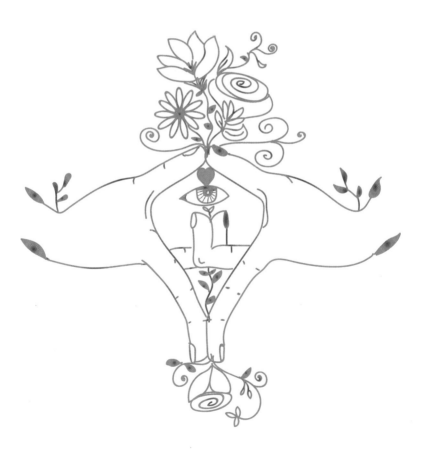

CHAPTER 2

Her Story of Yoni Steaming

Despite its relatively new emergence in the Western world, it appears that women have known about using heat, steam and herbs for vaginal health since antiquity. Vaginal steam bathing is an ancient healing practice that has been used for thousands of years to promote healing, balance and wellbeing for the reproductive organs.

Dr Rosita Arvigo, the founder of the Arvigo Techniques of Maya Abdominal Therapy®, spent decades studying the technique with Mayan women who use this natural remedy for any aspect of uterine pathology. Vaginal steaming is as popular in Mayan culture as drinking herbal tea is in Western culture. When a woman complained of any menstrual issue, she would be asked, 'Have you done your steam bath?' in the same way we would say, 'Have you drunk enough water?'

Traditional Korean healers used this method and called it *chai-yok*. They understood that yoni steaming increased blood circulation and relaxed the pelvic floor muscles. In Chinese Medicine it is used to relieve stagnation in the body and in Far Eastern Medicine to increase blood circulation and relax the pelvic floor muscles.

In ancient Greece, it was called 'vaginal fumigation'. Women heated a jar full of herbs and other carefully chosen ingredients and placed them into a hole dug in the ground. The top of the jar was firmly sealed except for a protruding reed that was inserted into the woman's vagina as she squatted over the hole. In this manner, the fumes from the jar were delivered internally.

In Africa, women would dig holes in the dirt and set fire to bark and native herbs placed within creating smoke that the women would crouch over. These practices were done with great ceremony before marriage after childbirth and also for medicinal uses.

In Indonesia, 'vaginal fogging' is an old Javanese custom whereby women were pampered in a secret location in a ceremony to beautify themselves prior to getting married. In a special ritual, a concoction of fragrant herbs including Betel Leaf was dissolved in hot water to emit a beautiful fragrant aroma. This mixture was used to steam and enhance a woman's yoni before the marriage night.

In ancient Egypt, women used the fragrant resins of Frankincense and Myrrh to cleanse their wombs by sitting on a low stool and allowing the scented resins to rise from below.

In Surinam, South America, women utilised steam as traditional medicine between menstrual cycles and after childbirth, abortions and miscarriages.

It also appears that vaginal steaming was evident in other parts of Asia, the Hawaiian Islands and Europe.

The *Trotula* is a fascinating medieval Italian text on women's medicine written in the 12th century. It describes how women were frequently 'afflicted in childbirth' and the diseases they subsequently suffered, especially around organs devoted to the work of Nature. The ingredients for a vaginal steam to bring back menses were listed as Ginger, Laurel Leaves and Savin Leaves (an evergreen bush). The instructions given were to pound the ingredients place them in a pot over live coals and have the woman sit upon a perforated seat. By allowing the smoke to be received through the lower members, the menses would return.

Vaginal fumigation was practiced in medieval times in an effort to treat the same reproductive ailments that women suffer from today: menstrual cramps, yeast infections and urinary tract infections. Herbs were mixed with water and boiled in a special container which had a long tube attached. Steam rose through the tube which was inserted into the vagina of the woman being treated. Thankfully today we have more hygienic and non-invasive methods.

Here in Australia, little is revealed about traditional Aboriginal women's business. From what we know, smoking and steaming have always been used as supportive indigenous rituals for birthing on country. Ritual cleansing, using steam produced from leaves and grasses, was traditionally practiced after childbirth by aboriginal women. The plants and leaves vary from state to state but the ceremony is the same. A pit is dug and leaves are placed over a small fire inside. As the fire dies down, the green plants give off their healing steam and the new mother is helped to sit or squat over the pit allowing the steam to act as a cleansing medicine.

In other places, at times of birth, women would squat over hot coals in a hole that was lined with Acacia Leaves and Sandalwood chips while water was splashed over the coals to produce steam. After birth, a woman would be helped to stand over a fire made at the base of an Ironwood tree, while water was thrown onto the fire to encourage smoke to enter her uterus. Women also squatted over a trough of burning Acacia to dry the vaginal lochia. Other types of Eucalyptus were used for smoking to prevent pain and bleeding after birth.

I acknowledge and honour the wisdom and knowledge of indigenous people around the world.

Evidently, yoni steaming has long been used as a healing medicine to provide relief for conditions associated with the womb centre and beyond, many of which remain heavily present in the 21st century.

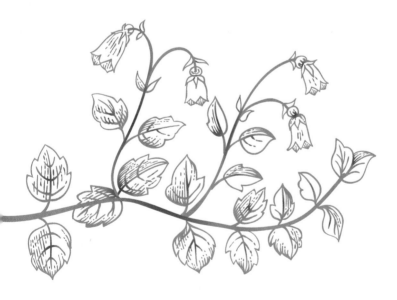

Chapter 3

Why Yoni Steam

The yoni is considered sacred not just in ancient Eastern civilisation but in other cultures as well. Images of yoni worship can be found in spiritual traditions across the world, recovered in ancient rock carvings and on figurines of shell and bone.

What our Ancestors Knew

In matriarchal times, goddess worship was practiced. Women were seen as manifestations of the Divine Mother, honoured and revered as goddesses. Their bodies, sexuality, fertility and sacred cycles were considered magic and powerful, the very embodiment of death and rebirth, of Life itself.

Over the centuries, women's sexuality was repressed and earth-based religions were replaced by patriarchy in league with the Church. Menstruation was considered to be Eve's curse. Women were deemed unclean and when their monthly cycle came around, were prohibited from the temples. The trauma of this oppression is evident to this day where many women consider their periods to be a nuisance—something to be ashamed of, hidden, or endured as a burden—and men still fear and shun women as being unclean.

In the 21st century, denigration of women and menstrual shame still exists. Insulting slang terms are commonly used to describe female genitalia and the menstrual cycle. I recently read about an interview with Cate Blanchett. She was asked where her moral compass existed in life. Without hesitation she answered boldly, 'in my vagina'. The interviewer was scandalised that not only had Cate used this *incendiary* term but that she had done so with absolute confidence, as if she was sitting on a special secret! It's unfortunate that mentioning this vital part of the female body in public is deemed as controversial.

Gratefully, this perception is changing as more and more women discover that they have an amazing spiritual apparatus built into their own bodies' psyches and womb space. There is huge opportunity for growth every month as a woman cycles with the moon and the tides' ebb and flow as she releases what she doesn't need physically and emotionally. As she learns how to harness this energy, she is able to manifest what she desires in life through letting go of ideas, relationships and beliefs that no longer serve her. The womb is the dreaming place of a woman: her birthplace of creation. Our foremothers knew this and honoured it by creating time to practice the ritual for cleansing and connection.

Yoni steaming is a wonderfully relaxing experience that will unwind your mind and soothe your body and soul. It is a beautiful ritual that opens and connects you to the deep feminine aspects of yourself that reside emotionally and spiritually in your womb. This practice creates space for you to focus on your womb centre and bring healing and love to an area that has been shamed and ignored—at best, dishonoured and at worst, abused.

Benefits of a Yoni Steam

- increases circulation to the whole reproductive system
- relieves menstrual cramps and irregular, painful and heavy periods. Lessens the occurrence of old, dark blood at beginning or end of your period
- reduces stress and regulates menstrual flow including irregular or absent menstrual cycles
- encourages the womb to her natural upright and open position for a smoother menstrual cycle
- detoxifies the womb and removes toxins from the body
- tones the pelvic floor and helps regulate the natural pH level of the womb
- stimulates production of hormones for uterine health
- aids in relieving vaginal or ovarian cysts and helps reduce uterine fibroids
- helps alleviate pain of endometriosis
- increases fertility, especially when combined with massage
- prepares your womb for a baby
- strengthens the womb and tones the vagina after birth
- reduces scarring from childbirth, such as episiotomy, vaginal tear or caesarean birth
- is soothing/healing after hysterectomy and laparoscopy

- encourages healing and tones the reproductive system after miscarriage or termination
- relieves symptoms of menopause and vaginal dryness
- helps with digestive issues
- helps with uterine prolapse
- on an emotional level, nourishes and supports the release of fears and beliefs that no longer serve you

This list is ever expansive. As more women discover this simple technique to improve their reproductive and emotional health and wellbeing, the benefits will be documented and the list will grow.

༄

Yoni steaming is powerful women's medicine.
I invite you to feel the truth of this in your body.

༄

WOMB WELLNESS

Womb wellness is a vital element of your health that affects you on every level. Your womb is the main gauge of your wellbeing. As a woman, you are a cyclical being. Your spiritual and emotional connection to your womb is amplified before and during your period. This is an ideal time to practice cleansing rituals such as yoni steaming.

How can you tell if your womb is healthy?

Your period is a reflection of your overall health. Every month you have the opportunity to look at your blood and gain insight into your health. Menstruation is not meant to be painful nor is it meant to feel like a major ordeal. It is important to note that when there is a build-up of old matter in the uterus, she has to work harder every month to do her job of shedding the endometrial lining. Having to work harder in order to function is what causes discomfort, fatigue and symptoms such as cramps and excessive bleeding.

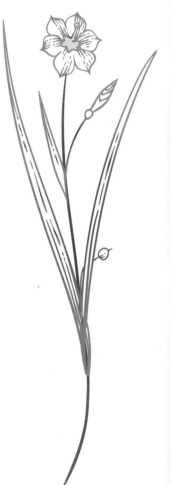

Your moon time should last for three to four days with little to no cramping. Menstrual blood should be ruby red. Brown blood at the beginning and/or end of your period is an indication of old blood from previous cycles.

Throughout every phase of your reproductive life, your womb tirelessly cycles with the moon and the tides. She waxes and wanes physically and emotionally every month. She also serves as the internal gauge of your welfare. When your womb is in pain, her symptoms are messages from the body that something is out of balance. If your womb is loved, honoured and respected what she feels on the inside will be reflected on the outside.

To put it bluntly: If something is up 'down there' then something is going on in your life that needs clearing.

Pay attention when your womb is in pain. She is trying to tell you something. Breathe deeply down to your womb space and ask her what she needs. She might have been trying to communicate with you for years.

Heal the womb and you heal the woman.

—Clare Spinx

SEASONS OF YOUR CYCLE

Your monthly cycle comes in four phases and corresponds with the seasons of the year, the four phases of the moon and the four facets of a woman's reproductive life. This is based on the twenty-eight-day cycle which is the average but not the norm for many women. Every cycle varies in length, but the one constant is that you will almost always ovulate fourteen days before menstruation. By applying what we know of the seasons, we can look at the menstrual cycle in a whole different way:

- Winter ~ Menstruation (days 1–7) ~ Crone
- Spring ~ Pre-Ovulation (days 7–14) ~ Maiden
- Summer ~ Ovulation (days 14–21) ~ Mother
- Autumn ~ Pre-Menstruation (days 21–28) ~ Wise woman

Your sacred menstrual code

Few of us were given the information we needed to be able to connect with our menstrual cycle in an empowering way. How would it be to think of your menstrual cycle as a sacred code embodied in your fabulous female body? As a woman, you are a cyclical being. When you rekindle a healthy relationship with your menstrual cycle, you will come to embrace the feminine wisdom that is literally embodied in you. It probably won't take place overnight. You may notice how you continue to push yourself even when your body is screaming out for rest, especially when you are bleeding. Eventually, you will learn when your energy levels are conducive with going for a job interview or running a marathon and when it would be best for you to stay at home with a good book. You can work with your menstrual cycle to manifest your desires. Imagine how your life might look if you honoured your energetic, sexual, emotional and spiritual needs every month.

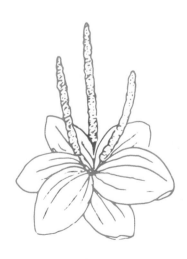

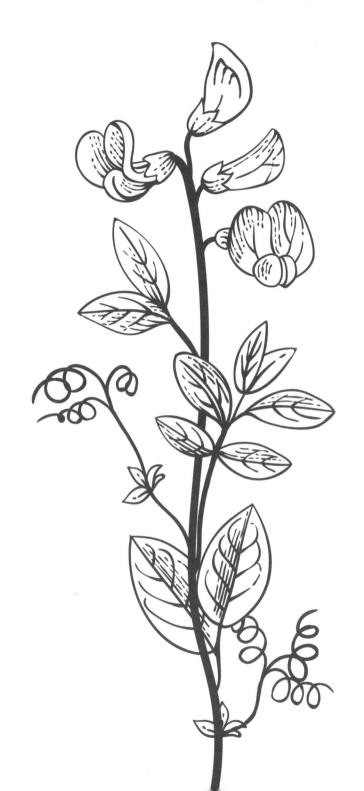

Chapter 4

When to Steam

Yoni steaming benefits women throughout all phases of their life and is especially helpful for the following experiences:

- menstrual cramps, hormone imbalance, fibroids, ovarian cysts, polycystic ovarian syndrome (PCOS) or endometriosis
- apprehension towards menstruation
- post-childbirth
- birth trauma, miscarriage, abortion or birth loss
- struggles with fertility challenges
- emotional trauma
- trauma from sexual abused, raped or injured
- perimenopause or menopause
- loss of libido and/or joie de vivre
- depression, anxiety, sadness or anger

- the desire for self-pampering and/or yoni pampering.
- the desire to try something new

Contraindications and Cautions

There are some circumstances in which yoni steaming is not suitable.

When **NOT** to Steam:

- when pregnant, or you think there is any possibility of pregnancy
- during menstruation
- when there is an active infection (cervical, uterine or ovarian)
- during a herpes outbreak or when open sores or blisters are present
- when a fever is present
- when burning or itchiness is present (as there is already an excess of heat)
- when there is any fresh, red bleeding
- when there is red, brown or pink spotting during a twenty-eight-day cycle
- when you spontaneously bleed between periods. If you have what is known as two periods in a month or have heavy spontaneous bleeding, you may have uterine fatigue and steaming is contraindicated
- Women who have short cycles of less than twenty-seven days should only do a mild vaginal steam for ten minutes. This is also because the uterus is fatigued and because steam increases circulation to the uterus it may bring on bleeding
- During a miscarriage steaming is contraindicated. It is recommended to wait until fresh bleeding has ceased

Can you steam if you have an IUD?

Some say yes while others say it may cause the IUD to dislodge and be expelled from the uterus. I say err on the side of caution. Have a short steam session for ten minutes without using an electric burner under your pot of herbs.

Can you steam in hot weather?

You may not feel like it. Consider using a sarong or a sheet as opposed to a blanket wrapped around you and steam for a shorter time. If you are a woman with hot flushes and/or have excess body heat, fifteen minutes might be enough for you.

Other considerations

Have a cup of tea or water bottle with you as a reminder to stay hydrated. Drink plenty of water afterwards.

I encourage you to tune into your body for the answers you seek. Once you get out of your thinking mind that is always trying to 'get it right', you will know intuitively whether yoni steaming is good for you on any one day during your cycle. You may simply feel too tired to set up your steam. This is a good indication to honour your tiredness. Consider at these times that having a nap or going to bed early might be a better option.

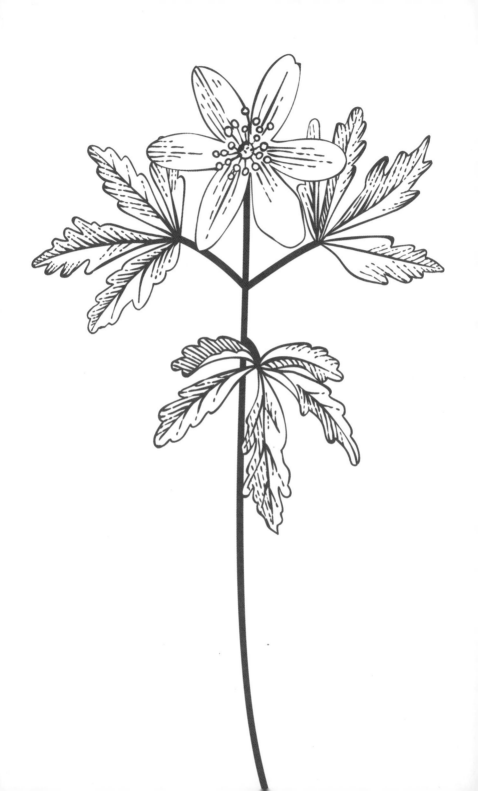

Chapter 5

How Does a Yoni Steam Work?

During a yoni steam, the warmth of the steam allows the vagina to soften open and become absorbent. The volatile oils and medicinal benefits of the plants are absorbed into the bloodstream through the vaginal tissues and ultimately reach the cervix uterus fallopian tubes and ovaries. The steam also warms and nourishes the internal membranes of the womb.

Not everyone agrees that the steam itself is able to enter the uterus. Some believe it is the warmth that heals as it creeps up through the vagina to the womb and into the heart. Practitioners agree, however, that a yoni steam will cleanse the uterine lining as evidenced by the cleansing reactions experienced by women when their next period comes.

The herbal formulas used in the steams stimulate pelvic circulation to cleanse, tone, nourish and heal the tissues as well as relax the muscles and deep fascia layers. The heat warms and nourishes the inside of the womb and expedites the release of waste and old, impacted endometrial lining. This may not be obvious at the time of steaming but may be evident at the next menses in the form of dark, thick blood, clots or residue. Do not be alarmed if this occurs. 'Better an empty apartment than a bad tenant', as Rosita Arvigo is fond of saying. Be gentle with yourself.

In time, sometimes even after only one or two sessions of steaming, your cycle will become easier. This will make your life sweeter in so many ways. You will feel healthier, have more energy and be able to connect with the wisdom of your menstrual cycle in a way that wasn't possible when you were in pain.

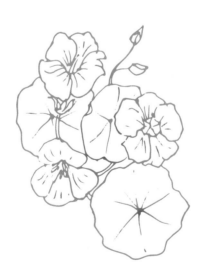

Chapter 6

Why Would You Steam Your Womb? That's Ridiculous

We have seen many naysayers who discount this practice as the latest alternative New Age health trend, or discount it as pseudo-science nonsense with no benefits. Some even go as far as saying the practice is detrimental to women's reproductive health, using the argument that the vagina is 'self-cleansing' and does not need to be detoxed, ever.

It is true that the vagina is self-cleaning, and it is important to recognise that yoni steaming is *not* supposed to clean your vulva or vagina.

It is also true that the benefit of vaginal steaming does not have the back-up of scientific or medical research (yet).

Why Would You Steam Your Womb? That's Ridiculous

45

Nor is there scientific research to say it doesn't work. Hopefully as this beautiful women's medicine becomes more widely practiced and women continue to share their healing stories with each other, it will become a recognised self-care modality that is part of women's health care.

I encourage you to try it for yourself. Conduct your own research. By taking responsibility for your own health you will be less inclined to give away your power to others. By taking the time to steam and meditate and go within, you will find out who you really are behind the conditioning and expectations of others. You will connect with your own womb intelligence. She only wants the very, very best for you. Connecting with yourself will empower you to naturally make choices more in alignment with who you really are. You will witness your self-love practices empower those around you.

Document your practice of yoni steaming and notice how it affects you mentally, emotionally and physically. Give yourself the gift of yoni steaming and the gift of connecting with your body. Cultivate a positive and loving relationship with your body and your menstrual cycle. Tune into your cyclical nature as a woman who is linked with the seasons as well as the moon and the tides. Notice the changes in your energy, creativity and moods throughout the month. Listen to your womb wisdom. Journal your insights and your dreams. Share with your sisters, your mother, your grandmother, aunties, cousins, neighbours and of course the men in your life!

୧ଡ଼ୱ

The soothing warmth of the steam will help you be compassionate with yourself.

୧ଡ଼ୱ

Chapter 7

Ingredients of a Yoni Steam

WATER

Water is sacred life giving and cleansing. We know it is one of the most essential nutrients required by all living things, the most abundant molecule in the body (our Earth and our bodies are made up of 70% water). The therapeutic qualities of water have been used to heal and relax the body and provide pain relief since time immemorial. People have always soaked in holy rivers underground caves natural hot springs and bathhouses.

Holy water is a crucial element in healing ceremonies throughout the world to cleanse purify and bless those who partake. Sanctified water is an integral part of Maya healing as it was and is recognised that blessing the water cleanses and purifies the body energetically and physically. The Maya understanding of disease is not limited to the physical. Like most traditional healing systems, the Mayans believe that disease stems from the soul and creates imbalances in the physical–emotional bodies that affect the *ch'ulel*, the Mayan word for 'chi' or 'inner vital energy'. Spiritual bathing is another potent form of emotional healing like yoni steaming using only the components of flowers, water, sunshine and prayer.

The Maya goddess of women and medicine

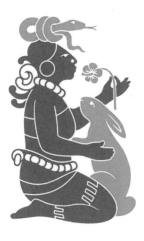

Where there is water, there is Ixchel, goddess of women the moon and medicine. She has been called 'the Heart of Water' and is connected to bodies of water, lakes, rivers and streams. She is most commonly depicted in her three main phases of Maiden, Mother and Crone. In her Crone phase she is depicted with a clay vessel of water. It is said that when she is in a good mood she pours blessings upon the earth, but when vexed she sends forth storms, floods and hurricanes. There are water goddesses associated with fertility and creation stories in every ancient culture connected with the sea, rivers, sacred springs and waterholes.

Through Dr Masaru Emoto's work we know that thoughts and emotions affect the molecular structure of water. Water listens. It is receptive to prayer and connects us to all that is. This means that your thoughts have a profound impact on your health. Programming the water you use for your yoni steam with loving thoughts and prayers raises the vibrations and will add a whole new dimension to your experience.

STEAM

Steam is powerful energy. It has always bubbled up out of hot spots in the earth. Steam generates electricity and can drive a boat across the ocean or a train over a mountain. When you heat water on the stove, the water molecules start bubbling around, becoming more and more energised until the volume of the steam becomes greater than the original volume of liquid. We have already seen how powerful water is. Now we see how extraordinary steam is!

Steam baths have been used to promote healing for thousands of years. Steam opens up the pores and releases toxins from the body. Steam therapy is recognised by Western medicine and is considered good for your heart and arteries. It is used for skin conditions, arthritis, allergies and hypertension. It makes sense that warm, nurturing steam will improve womb health.

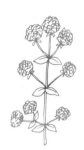

HERBS

Mother Nature bestows many gifts. Some of her most beautiful offerings come in the guise of flowers and herbs. The healing power of flowers is so potent that even gazing at their beauty brings joy. There are particular flowers that possess phytochemicals that have anti-inflammatory, antibacterial and cardiovascular properties that benefit the body. For example: the sunny Golden/Orange Calendula, a common ingredient in yoni steams, contains glycosides that are anti-inflammatory, antiviral and anticarcinogenic.

꧁꧂

It is said there is a herb to cure every ailment.

꧁꧂

When you grow the herbs in your own garden you work in companionship with Mother Nature and her nature spirits. They are delighted that you are accessing the healing gifts of the earth and you will be guided to the plants that have the healing properties that your body needs. Tuning into their unique medicine you can drink herbs as teas take them as tinctures and steam with them too. Remember to choose and gather the flowers and herbs for your yoni steam with gratitude and appreciation.

These three elements combined with positive intentions create a powerful healing force that is available for you to soothe and address pain congestion and imbalance in the reproductive system, both on a physical and energetic level.

CHAPTER 8

How to do a Yoni Steam at Home

To do a yoni steam at home, you will need:

- yoni seat, stool or chair, strong enough to bear your weight
- Slow cooker with porcelain inner bowl OR a stainless steel pot to be heated on your stove top or electric burner
- eight cups of (filtered) water
- fresh or dried herbs
- a warm blanket or cloak that goes all the way to the floor to keep the heat in

Traditionally, herbs are gathered with prayer and intention. The Maya offered prayers nine times to the Maya spirits. They believed that without prayer the steaming would be ineffective. You may offer your devotions to whomever you pray to. Choose herbs that 'speak' to you. In other words, herbs you love! Thank them for their beauty and generosity. Enjoy the nature spirits that abound. This will enhance your spiritual experience.

༄

Mother Nature provides you with everything you need to heal.

༄

YOUR YONI THRONE

There are many versions of yoni thrones on the market. Some look like birthing stools while other versions are boxed in with an opening for you to sit over. DIY options include a camping toilet seat, a chair with a hole cut out of the base or a wooden garden chair with slats. Please make sure your yoni seat is sturdy and able to hold your weight. It is very important it does not collapse underneath you.

Setting up Your Steam

Find a private spot where you will not be disturbed. You will need an electrical socket if using a slow cooker. Cleanse the area with Sage or Copal. Create your own yoni healing space by laying down a beautiful rug or cloth to sit on. This is where you will sit in quiet reverence.

You may have a goddess figure some oracle cards for guidance or wish to arrange your favourite crystals or vase of flowers.

Light a candle.

Begin by placing one hand on your heart and one hand on your womb.

Then:

- Set loving and healing intentions for your steam session.

- Give thanks for your herbs and the water.

- If using a saucepan or stainless-steel pot on a stove, add herbs to the water, bring to the boil and simmer for ten minutes. Carefully carry the pot and place it under your yoni seat. Remove the lid, and check the temperature with your hand.

- For a longer session use your slow cooker or saucepan on a burner. Place under seat add boiling water, then the herbs. Switch to 'cook' for ten minutes. Turn to OFF when you are ready to begin. Adjust temperature if steam cools down.

- Be mindful that the temperature of the steam should feel pleasant and soothing—not too hot, not too cold. You may need to adjust the heat during your session.

- Wrap yourself in your blanket.

- Take your time sitting over the steam. Always be mindful that you are lowering your vulva over steaming vapour. Be careful not to burn yourself. Stand up and wait for a few minutes to let the steam cool down if it feels too hot.
- Wear woolly socks to keep your feet warm.
- Smell the fragrance of your herbs and flowers.
- Invite the steam in.
- Enjoy this quiet, sacred time to yourself. Turn your attention inwards. Breathe slowly and deeply into your womb space. Listen to the whispers of your inner self.

Ask yourself:

- What does your womb wish to say to you?
- What has she been trying to tell you for years perhaps?

Pay attention.

WARNINGS

NEVER use essential oils in vaginal steams. They are too strong for the soft and delicate tissues of your yoni. Nor should the recommended herbs for vaginal steams be taken internally as the properties of herbs work differently when taken internally.

REMOVE any genital piercings. The metal will heat up and may burn you.

Chapter 9

What to Expect from a Yoni Steam

Session Duration

Session duration should be approximately twenty-thirty minutes. By the time the herbs have released their healing properties, most women feel like they have had long enough to absorb them. Longer sessions are advised for chronic conditions under guidance from a qualified practitioner. Please tune in and listen to your body and your womb.

Steaming is not a practice that endorses more is better. If your menstrual cycle is less than twenty-eight days, it is recommended that you steam for only ten minutes. If you have a more chronic ailment like endometriosis, fibroids or cysts, your steam session may be longer. If one of these conditions is present, please seek the guidance of an Arvigo® practitioner or a vaginal steam therapist for support.

Do not overheat yourself. Dry yourself off when you have finished. Stay warm and avoid cool drafts after your steam.

Try to plan your steam for a not-so-busy day!

$\backslash$ை

Remember to return the water and your herbs to the garden. Give thanks to Mother Earth for the healing blessings of the plants.

$\backslash$ை

Breathe deeply and slowly into your womb centre during your steam. Do not carry or use your mobile phone. Instead, use this time to meditate or pray. There are guided womb meditations that you may like to listen to (see Resources for a list of guided meditations). This is an opportunity to be present and tune into your womb's inner voice. What does she want you to hear? What has she been trying to tell you? Trust the guidance you receive.

After your Steam

You may feel lightheaded, sleepy, euphoric or emotional. Because of the detoxifying effects of the steam, you might feel tired and emotional. You might cry. It is important to take time to rest after your steam.

You might notice some slight cramping and vaginal discharge after your steam. This is normal. There are likely to be changes in your next menstrual cycle. Your next period might come early. The herbs have a powerful effect on the uterus and may dislodge old encrusted material from the inside lining of the endometrium.

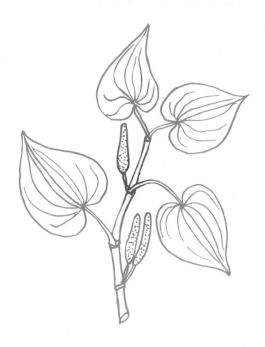

Don't be alarmed if you release dark blood, clots and old residual matter that looks like coffee grounds. Your bleeding may be heavier than usual for a day or two. You might experience cramping as your womb works hard to release the old stuff. Consider that your body might have been storing this old residue for years as a result of incomplete bleeding. In time, your bleeding will become lighter and you may even find yourself looking forward to your menstrual period.

ᘒ

Keeping warm is at the heart of traditional women's medicine across the world. Heat is medicine for a woman's body. It supports opening and release, whereas cold causes contraction.

ᘒ

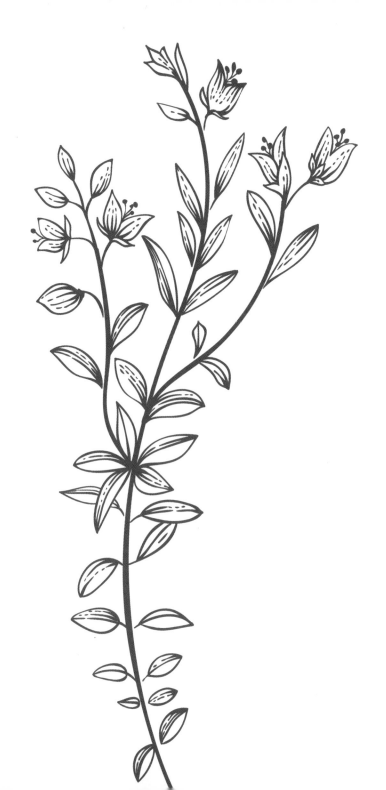

Chapter 10

How Often and When You Should Steam

Whether you are steaming for health concerns or simply for your reproductive wellbeing will determine the time and frequency of your steams. As more comprehensive knowledge is gathered about the properties of the herbs and the effects of steaming, we will see more documented and proven protocols for different ailments. For now, it is suggested that if you suffer from painful periods you may steam two to three times in the week before you bleed and once after your cycle ends to fully flush out your womb.

For fertility you may steam once before and once after your period and twice more leading up to ovulation.

Do not steam after ovulation if there is any possibility of pregnancy. If your period comes you can resume steaming. Expect to steam for three months before seeing results knowing that you will be cleansing and improving your uterine lining in readiness for conception.

For womb health and vitality steam in the last week of your cycle and again at the beginning of the next cycle when you have stopped bleeding. You might like to steam once a week for each week of your menstrual cycle unless you are trying to conceive.

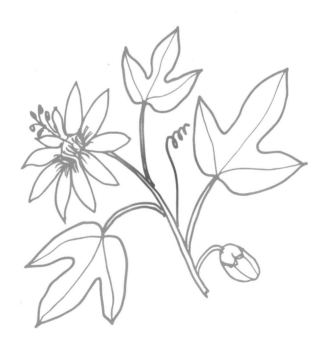

Chapter 11

During a Steam

Breathe Down to Your Womb While You Steam

Deep belly breathing is so good for you and your womb! Conscious deep breathing can be done anytime (not just while you steam). Your womb will respond gladly, especially if you make it a regular practice. Your life will begin to transform as you create more space in your lungs and chest allowing more oxygen and life force energy to flow into your womb.

Sigh. Say Aaaaaaaaaah. Feel the vibrations resounding in your womb space and let the sound help to release pent up emotions. Listening to music is also calming while you steam.

Meditate While You Steam

Focus on your breath. Visualise warm, healing light flowing in from your soul chakra above your head down into your womb. Use your imagination to either see in your mind's eye or feel this flow of light energy running down your body. Picture this energy releasing any pain or blockages in your womb with ease and grace, gently scrubbing away any leftover sorrow or lingering sadness. You may have to practice this exercise, though try not to let it feel arduous. If you do not see or feel anything, that's OK too.

Breathe in positive energy and visualise your womb filling with gladness, joy and inspiration for new projects. This is a great practice to do before your period begins each month.

Yoni Steam Affirmations

- My body is healthy.
- My womb is healthy.
- I trust my womb.
- I love my yoni.
- I welcome healing energy into my womb space.
- I let go of what no longer serves me.

What would you like to add here?

....

....

....

....

Cup of Tea with Your Steam

There are many herbs known to nourish your uterus, support its tone and function and improve uterine health for fertility, conception and implantation. Whether you are preparing for pregnancy or just want to be healthier herbal teas can cleanse your uterus while also removing excess hormones and toxins in the liver. Many of them taste good as a tea too. Three herbs with particularly supportive qualities are Red Raspberry Leaves, Nettle Leaves and Red Clover.

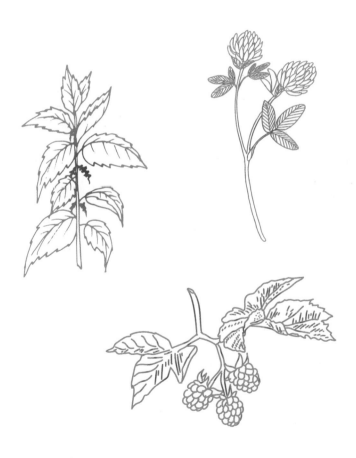

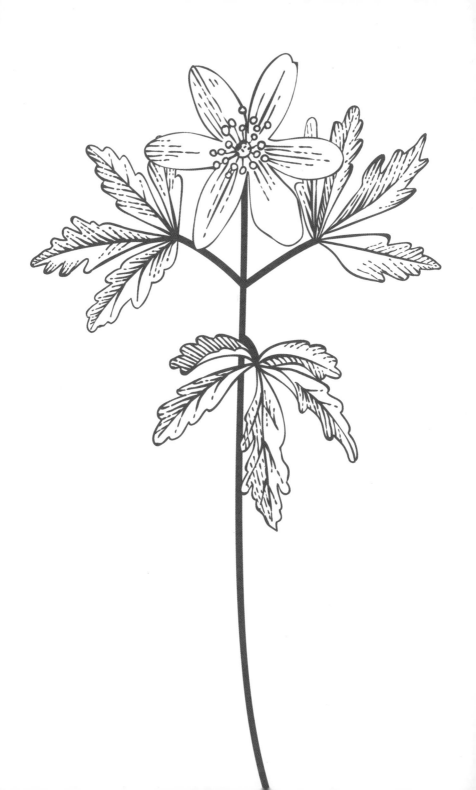

CHAPTER 12

Postpartum Benefits of Yoni Steaming

Vaginal steaming has long been used by midwives around the globe for postpartum healing. During pregnancy the uterus stretches to nine times its size. Birth complications, difficult births and lack of breastfeeding may prevent the uterus from returning to its pre-pregnancy size and tone. Vaginal steaming is a great way to increase circulation, reduce bloating and tone the whole pelvic area. It also helps to prevent a prolapsed uterus.

For many generations before us, traditional midwives and birth attendants around the world have assisted women to steam after the birth of their baby. The soothing warmth of the steam helps to cleanse the womb, heal the placental site and relieve uterine pain and cramps. Keeping warm is at the heart of traditional practices following birth across the cultures. Doing a yoni steam postpartum brings nourishing heat to support the body to release lochia, fluids and any remnants of placental tissue. This will help the womb to involute back to pre-pregnancy size. Postpartum steaming will cleanse and disinfect stitches and perineal tears and help with the healing of haemorrhoids. It has also been shown to help lose weight gained through pregnancy.

In Central America, three days after birth the new Mayan mother sat over a round opening in a stone bench and was given a yoni steam with nine herbs. In Haiti, it has been traditional for women to do a vaginal stream with herbs every day for two weeks after birth to tone and heal the pelvic floor and clean out the uterus.

Now there are different opinions as to when and how often you should steam after birth. Some say you should wait until bleeding has finished. Others say you can steam within two or three days after giving birth. Another suggestion is to steam daily or three times a week for a month to facilitate healing and toning of the uterus. Under guidance, some women steam three days in a row within the first nine days and then three times a week for a month.

This ancient, postnatal womb medicine is having a renaissance though it may be something your midwife is not familiar with. You might have to be the one to teach her about this practice. Come up with a plan and document your results knowing that your experience and personal research will help many, many women in the future. Hopefully the emerging new profession and services of postnatal doulas will see the influx of yoni steaming being brought to the new mama in her own home.

Keli Gaza, founder of Steamy Chick, steamed for thirty minutes for thirty days after the birth of her babies, beginning in the second week as part of her postnatal self-care routine. She reported that her lochia was all expelled quickly and her vaginal tissues shrank back to normal. Her uterine prolapse corrected itself and her haemorrhoids were cured (see Resources).

Astrid, a new mother who sustained a perineal tear after giving birth to Noah, when he was seven months old said, 'I love how I can feel everything healing while I meditate and relax'. Another new mama found relief from postpartum haemorrhoids due to the soothing and comforting warmth of the steam.

Perineal Injury/Episiotomy

To heal, soften and cleanse the tissues after stitches from a perineal tear or episiotomy, a yoni steam will help speed up the healing process and provide soothing warmth and comfort.

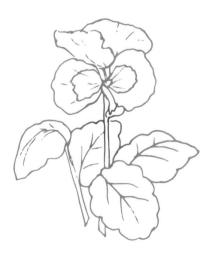

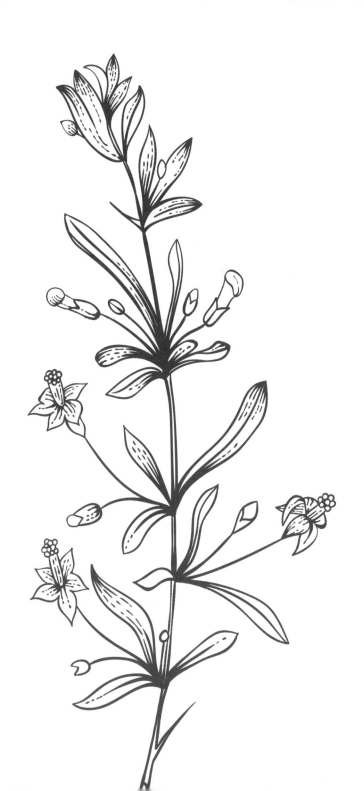

CHAPTER 13

Steaming for all Stages of a Woman's Life

Comforting, warming heat combined with stimulating herbs increases circulation and blood flow to your pelvis and reproductive organs. This is helpful for all the stages of your reproductive life.

MENARCHE

Young girls over the age of thirteen may steam under the guidance of a practitioner. A mother who has learnt to steam is in the ideal position to share this with her teenage daughter, especially if she suffers from physical and emotional discomfort prior to her period. This is also the ideal time to celebrate her daughter's menarche and support her to value her period as a positive experience. A young girl needs to only steam for only ten minutes using gentle herbs.

The Reproductive Years

Prevention is better than cure. Yoni steaming is a safe, effective method for women to maintain menstrual and hormonal health throughout their reproductive years. Even if you have a healthy stress-free cycle, you can still have a vaginal steam. Most women take the time to moisturise their hair, face and lips on a daily basis. Why not consider yoni steaming as a nurturing monthly self-care practice? You can steam twice a month for maintenance and relaxation: once before your period and once afterwards. Enjoy making this part of your self-care routine.

For Period Problems

Until recently, the symptoms of painful cramps, emotional ups and downs, headaches, just to name a few, have been viewed as normal and women have been expected to endure pain every month as a part of being a woman. When periods begin with brown blood it is an indication that the endometrial lining has not been completely cleansed from the previous cycle. If it ends with brown this may be a sign that the womb has not fully flushed out during the current cycle. If your period begins with brown, steam in the days before your period is due. If it ends with brown, steam after you have finished bleeding.

Postpartum

Vaginal steaming has been used by midwives in the postpartum period to provide warmth, promote healing of the placental site and encourage the organs to return to their pre-pregnancy position.

Perimenopause

It is important for your uterus to fully release all blood, fluids and any residue in the months, possibly years, leading up to menopause. Yoni steams will help balance your hormones and empty out the uterus completely before bleeding ceases.

When your cycle begins to change and slow down, steaming will stimulate circulation and support your womb to release, while nourishing a deep connection to the awakening wise woman within you. This is a time of transition and transformation to be celebrated, not feared. This is a good time to do something radical like steaming your yoni! Using vaginal steams during your perimenopausal years will help cleanse and fully release blood and fluids before your cycles finish and will help settle your hormones.

Menopause

For wise women who no longer bleed, you may steam a few times a year for maintenance. Some say try it on the full moon while others say the new moon. Follow your intuition. During this time of great transition, the female hormones oestrogen and progesterone fluctuate and decline bringing unwelcome symptoms such as hot flushes, vaginal dryness and loss of libido. This is a challenging time of a woman's life that has been feared and demonised rather than seeing it as a time of great personal power and transformation. A yoni steam will give you time for inner reflection and connection to your ageing female body that is by no means past her prime. You may no longer be able to reproduce but you can start a new career, travel, fulfil lifelong dreams and enjoy life to the full with a renewed sense of self and peace of mind. Caution: Having said all that, if you experience hot flushes, it may not be ideal for you to steam.

The Queen Phase

The Maiden, Mother and Crone represent the three major stages of a woman's life. The Maiden represents the creator, the Mother the nurturer and the Crone the wise woman. In the 21st century women live longer and experience greater health and vitality in their later years. Because the Crone is often negatively portrayed as old and gnarly, women have rejected this archetype and have embraced the new version of the Queen or the Enchantress. Being able to create a yoni steam ritual during this major transition of life will nurture and strengthen a deep connection to your womb space. It will foster a meditative practice that draws your attention naturally inwards to your belly and your womb intuition. Here you can reflect on what is it that calls you. What will bring you fulfilment and satisfaction at this transformative time.

ᘻ

Breathe deeply down to your womb.
Let go what no longer serves you.

ᘻ

Note: Women who have not bled for years have reported a cleansing release of fluids and even blood after doing a yoni steam. This does not mean that the menstrual cycle has resumed.

POST-MENOPAUSE

Menopause is when one year has passed since your final bleed. Send lots of love and gratitude down to your womb for the tireless labour she has done for you every month since you began menstruating. You may not have appreciated this labour and your relationship with your womb may have been fraught with anxiety. It's never too late to appreciate her. She still remains in your pelvic bowl physically, and also energetically if she is gone from your body. Steaming will provide physical and emotional sustenance at this time as well as promoting healthy circulation and hormonal balance.

The fragrant herbs and warmth of the steam support circulation and blood flow to your pelvis and keep your pelvic floor toned and relaxed. Steaming four times a year or once for every season may be another guide for post-menopausal steaming. There are a number of symptoms that may arise in this stage.

VAGINAL DRYNESS

Vaginal dryness, discomfort, and pain during intercourse are other distressing but common symptoms of menopause. Warming steam and moisturising herbs such as Marshmallow, Nettles, Mint and Calendula will warm up and revitalise the vaginal tissues.

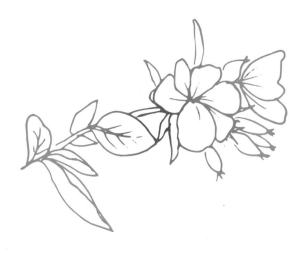

Painful sex

Unfortunately, this is often linked with vaginal dryness. Declining oestrogen levels and declining mucus production mean less vaginal lubrication and sensitive constricted and irritable vaginal walls. Many women experience pain during intercourse but like other female complaints, it is not a subject that is openly talked about. The yoni steam offers a pleasurable method to soften, lubricate and relax the tissues.

Lost libido

Loss of sexual desire may be attributed to declining progesterone levels at this time. Hot flushes and night sweats (from lowered oestrogen levels) may decrease feelings of sexiness and lack of lubrication can lead to painful sex. Vaginal steaming may prove to be a fun way to become lubricated and juicy again. There is also a pleasant rumour that it promotes better orgasms. Orgasms mean more oxytocin, feelings of love and connection, and increased circulation to your womb.

Prolapse

Steaming brings nourishment and circulation to the pelvic floor and perineum. Whether it is a prolapse from a recent birth or from one decades ago, steaming will improve and tone the muscles of the perineum. Supportive modalities such as the Arvigo Techniques of Maya Abdominal Therapy® and pelvic physiotherapy will also assist.

Cervical Dysplasia

Cervical dysplasia is a precancerous condition in which abnormal cell growth occurs on the surface lining of the cervix. See Kate's account in the Testimonials section.

Healing from Past Relationships

Women may use yoni steaming to cleanse themselves of unwanted memories of past partners, sexual abuse or even rape. Feelings of violation may stay with a woman for decades. The gentle and soothing yoni steam offers the opportunity to cleanse, heal and let go of any residual anger, sadness or shame associated with the trauma.

Every time you are intimate with your partner you allow them into your body. This leaves an imprint and an energy signature upon your womb and sexual organs. When a relationship or pregnancy ends, you are left with the remnants of that experience as energy imprinted within you. Each intimate relationship you have takes up space within your womb and energy body. If the relationship is not healthy this energy can build up become stagnant and cause disharmony within you.

Likewise, miscarriages and abortions have a similar effect. Energy imprints are left behind like tiny scars. When you lose a baby through miscarriage or if you have had an abortion, the energy stays with you in much the same way as a partner's energy stays with you. These traumatic events are held in your womb and sacral chakra and may leave you with emotional scars as unresolved emotions can deeply affect your ability to move on or conceive again in the future. A yoni steam will help you to cleanse and purify your body and soul from shame, guilt and the past. This may take time so please be gentle with yourself.

ﮩ

Give Mother Nature just half a chance.
She has a miracle in store for everyone.

—Rosita Arvigo, DN

ﮩ

Chapter 14

Medicinal Properties of Flowers and Herbs

Which Herbs to Use

Yoni steaming provides a direct conduit for herb and plant medicine to penetrate the womb. When boiled and simmered, herbs release their unique medicine and can be used to treat chronic infections, menstrual and reproductive disorders and promote fertility. Herbs with strong smells ensure a higher volatile oil content and therefore provide more physical medicine. Mayan healers and midwives used Oregano, Basil, Marigold, Rosemary, Burdock Leaves, Motherwort, St John's Wort,

Chamomile, Damiana, Plantain, Horsetail, Rose Petals, Red Clover, Yarrow, Dandelion and Yellow Dock, amongst others. The good news is that nearly all these herbs grow well in many states of Australia.

GROWING HERBS IN YOUR BACKYARD

I am blessed to live in Northern New South Wales, Australia, where most herbs grow well in my garden. It is best to find out what herbs will grow in your own local area or in pots on your veranda. They say herbs grow where they are most needed. Get to know your herbal allies and experiment with using them in your steams. Many gardens have Rose, Rosemary, and Lavender bushes. You might have Basil growing as a companion plant for your tomatoes. Oregano is easy to grow in many climates. All of these beautiful culinary herbs have beneficial healing properties for womb healing. Gardening itself is good for your soul. You don't have to have a green thumb to benefit from being outside with the fresh air and nature spirits.

For yoni steams, the herbs can be used fresh if available or dried. Always choose organic or wild plants when possible to eliminate chemicals from pesticides or herbicides disturbing the purity of your steam. You can use one herb at a time or try a combination. The benefit of a blend is that you combine the healing properties and actions of several herbs at once.

Shakti Whispers Herb Blend – Mild Blend

A gentle blend suitable for first-time steam sessions.

- ½ tsp Motherwort
- ½ tsp Lavender
- 2 tsp Nettle
- 2 tsp Mint
- 1.5 litres boiling water

Womb Blessing Blend – for Meditation and Quiet Reflection

- Small handful of Rose Petals
- 1 tsp Lion's Tail
- 1tsp Calendula
- 1 tsp Lavender
- ½ tsp Motherwort
- 1 tsp Rosemary
- 1.5 litres boiling water

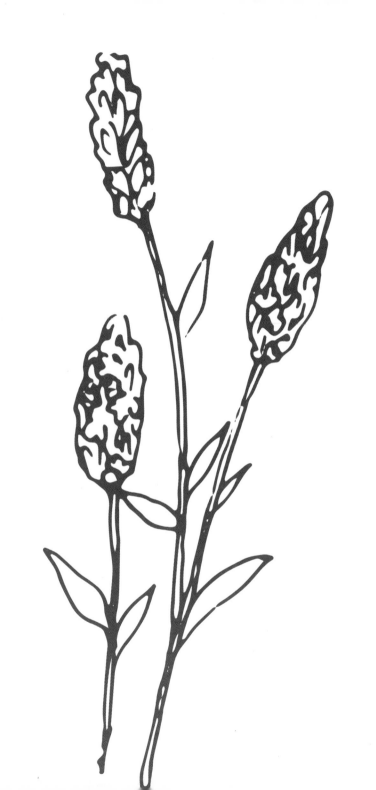

CHAPTER 15

Healing Herbs

Always ask the herbs for help with what you wish to heal.

It is important to understand the properties of the herbs and the effect they will have on your body when you add them to a steaming blend. Are they cooling? Moisturising? Do they increase circulation? Do they have antibacterial properties? Are they drying? A herb like Lavender might be beautiful for a woman with painful period cramps but too drying for a menopausal woman. The presenting symptoms of a woman will determine which combination of herbs will work for specific ailments. It is also necessary to look at her menstrual cycle in order to correctly formulate a unique blend. The herbs prescribed by a Traditional Chinese Medicine practitioner may provide additional support for reproductive issues.

BASIL

Spiritually cleansing, this herb is known to bring on the return of absent menses. Reduces menstrual cramps. Antibacterial. Blesses the woman receiving its properties.

CALENDULA

This beautiful colourful herb brings joy, vitality and healing to the womb. Its volatile oils heal wounds and scar tissue and it is very gentle on the delicate skin of the vulva. It is known to activate lymph flow and alleviate fungal and bacterial infections.

CHAMOMILE

Relaxing and calming, Chamomile has anti-inflammatory properties and is soothing to the vaginal tissues.

LAVENDER

Lavender is a gentle and relaxing herb that alleviates anxiety and calms the spirit, mind and body. Its beautiful purple flowers are antibacterial, antiviral and astringent. It nourishes the nervous system and has an antispasmodic effect on the uterus (eases cramps). It is also emollient and very soothing to irritated tissues. However, it is quite drying so is not recommended for menopause. It is also not a herb of choice if trying to conceive.

Lemon Balm

Lemon Balm is another soothing and uplifting herb that helps reduce yoni itchiness. It smells delightful when its scented volatile oils are released. It is also delicious to enjoy as a herbal tea while you steam.

Lemon Myrtle

This beautiful Australian native has powerful antiseptic and antiviral properties. The leaves are extremely beneficial for yoni steaming. Due to its drying nature you only need a tiny amount. It smells wonderful too. Drunk as a tea (while you steam) the leaves of the Lemon Myrtle can be used to treat colds and allergies and to boost the immune system.

Lemon Verbena

Calming and astringent with a distinctive citrus smell. Good for treating yeast infections. Reduces menstrual cramps and hot flushes. Lovely to drink as a fragrant herbal tea while you steam.

Leonotis Leonurus

This beautiful herb is a tonic to the eye due to its vibrant orange flowers as well as being a valuable tonic for the reproductive system. It has been used to treat premenstrual symptoms, regulate the menstrual cycle and bring on delayed menses.

MARIGOLD

Like Calendula, this cheerful flower will gladden your heart as well as your yoni. It cleanses and soothes and helps to heal vaginal tissues after birth.

MARSHMALLOW

The flowers of Marshmallow are moisturising and cooling and a beautiful addition to your steam. Marshmallow Root is anti-inflammatory and good for vaginal dryness and menstrual cramps.

MINT

The smell of Mint drifting up from your steam pot will lift your spirit, calm your mind and moisturise your vaginal tissues. Grown abundantly in many gardens, it is a mild blood tonic and good for menopause.

MOTHERWORT

Motherwort is known as the healer of the heart of the womb. It cleanses, nourishes and tones the womb and increases circulation to the whole pelvis. It is believed to encourage the breakdown of clots, fibroids and polyps. Eases menstrual cramps and increases menstrual flow by relaxing the uterine muscles. Beneficial for emotional healing and postpartum support.

MUGWORT

Mugwort has long been known to have an affinity with womb health. It has powerful circulatory properties, cleanses physically and spiritually and helps bring on menses. According to Traditional Chinese Medicine, the word 'uterus' translates as 'womb palace' and great respect is given to its ability to both store and release blood every month. TCM also gives credence to vaginal steaming as a way of helping energy to flow in and out of the womb. Herbs with strong smells ensure a higher volatile oil content and therefore provide more physical medicine. This is why Mugwort is so well used. As well as warming and dispelling dampness in the womb, Mugwort is attributed to having magical powers that protect one from evil spirits and is a beneficial herb to heal sexual trauma. It is not recommended to use Mugwort while breastfeeding.

Nettle

Nourishing, moisturising and is a superb blood tonic.

Oregano

Oregano is easy to grow the world over and is one of the best herbs for steams. Antiseptic and antibacterial, it helps prevent infections. As a uterine stimulant, it is an excellent herb to bring on menses and to increase low, inadequate menstrual flow.

Red Clover

These friendly little blooms balance hormones, increase blood circulation to the womb and support healthy cervical mucous. Optimises fertility. Beneficial for menstrual cramps.

Red Raspberry Leaf

Red Raspberry Leaf provides gentle medicine for the womb. Well known as a superb uterine tonic, the properties in Red Raspberry Leaf relax and tone the uterus. It is healing for post-surgery, heavy menstrual bleeding and reproductive ailments such as cysts, fibroids, endometriosis and prolapse. It has been long used to prepare the uterus for labour and birth by drinking as a tea. Now you can use it in your yoni steam in the postpartum period.

Rosemary

This beautiful aromatic herb has always been associated with protection. Antiseptic, cleansing and purifying, it is helpful to treat bacterial infection. Rosemary loves the womb. It increases circulation to the pelvis, can bring on menses and will clear out old blood, fluids and anything that is no longer needed. Known to promote wound healing, Rosemary will also help soothe emotional wounds and trauma.

Rose petals

Relaxing and uplifting, the beautiful Rose Petals act as a gentle astringent for internal tissues. They increase self-love and help to releases stuck emotions. Traditional midwife's remedy to reduce uterine haemorrhage. Lovely for post-menopausal steams.

Sage/White Sage

Sage is astringent and spiritually cleansing. It releases emotional and energetic blockages and helps you get in touch with your spirit guides. You only need a small amount in your steam to benefit from its disinfecting properties.

Thyme

Thyme is another great cleansing and antiseptic herb that helps to let go of melancholy. Great as an immune booster and also reported to be an aphrodisiac.

Wormwood

Wormwood is good for immunity. It is known for its antimicrobial properties and its sedative and detoxing effects on the womb.

Yarrow

Yarrow is a mystical herb that is beneficial for overall uterine health. Like a tuning fork it scans the womb's energy field and does what the womb needs. Known as the healer of the menstrual cycle its properties are astringent, cleansing and antibacterial. It is one of the best herbs to stop heavy bleeding due to fibroids. Also good for infections and for treating ovarian cysts.

Heart and Soul Blend

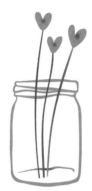

- 3–4 Rose Petals
- 1 tsp Mugwort
- 1 tsp Lion's Tail
- 1 tsp Calendula
- ½ tsp Lavender
- ½ tsp Rosemary
- 1 tsp Lemon Balm
- 1.5 litres of boiling water

NOTE: A reminder not to use essential oils in your vaginal steam. The oils are too strong for your delicate genital tissues.

৩৩

Herbs are healing and regenerative,
but they have no hands.

—Rosita Arvigo, DN

৩৩

CHAPTER 16

Steaming Wisdom

Give yourself time to absorb the healing medicine and allow your womb to integrate the effects of the steam. Healing energy will unwind and unravel tension as it flows through your body. The yoni steam is a sacred ritual and is most beneficial when recognised and acknowledged as such. It is best to perform your yoni steam when you have adequate time to appreciate and integrate the experience. By doing your yoni steam at night you can have a warm bath afterwards and go straight to bed. After a yoni steam, pay attention to your dreams.

CRYSTAL-INFUSED YONI STEAM

We have already spoken about the power of thought, prayers and setting intentions while preparing your yoni steam. You can also program the water and enhance your steam by adding crystals. This will change the molecular structure of the water and amplify the healing benefits and potency of the herbal steam.

There are several gemstones and crystals that may enhance the healing effects of the herbs in your yoni steam. Using Quartz is a powerful way to program your yoni steam with beneficial energy. Rose Quartz is well known for its soft, soothing energy of unconditional love. Other feminine healing stones are Adventurine, Moonstone and Carnelian. You can mix the crystals with your herbs in a container beforehand so their properties can be absorbed.

To prepare your crystal-infused yoni steam

Place your crystals in a bowl of water and allow them to sit in the sunlight or moonlight for several hours. This is an opportune time for you to take a moment to pray over the water and set your intentions. Use the water to prepare your yoni steam as per usual. You may also combine the crystals with your herbs as you prepare them over the heat. Remember to return the water, herbs and crystals back to the earth or into a body of water with gratitude after your steam. Or you might prefer to retrieve your crystals to use again.

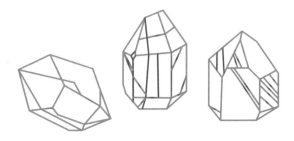

Crystal Heart and Soul Blend

- ½ tsp Lavender
- ½ tsp Marigold
- ½ tsp Mugwort
- 1 tsp Raspberry Leaves
- 1 tsp Red Rose Petals
- 1tsp Lemon Balm
- ½ tsp Rosemary
- ½ tsp Basil
- ½ tsp each Rose Quartz, Carnelian and Citrine chips
- 1.5 litres boiling water

Alternatives to Using Herbs in Your Steam

If you are unable to access herbs, for example if you are travelling or don't have any herbs at home or in the garden, there are alternatives.

Steam with Salt

Salt is antibacterial, rich in minerals and helps to regulate blood flow as well as balance your pH. Use natural, unprocessed salt such as Himalayan or sea salt.

- ½ tsp salt
- 1.5 litres boiling water

Apple Cider Vinegar

- ¼ cup Apple Cider Vinegar
- 1.5 litres boiling water

Steam with H₂O

We know the healing effects of steam. If you have no access to herbs, you can steam with water only.

Female Ailments and Herbal Formulas

To tone and strengthen the reproductive and urinary organs: Red Raspberry Leaf, Rosemary and Motherwort.

Vaginal dryness: Marshmallow, Calendula, Chamomile, Red Clover and Mugwort.

Painful menstrual cramps: Motherwort, Basil, Lavender, Lemon Verbena, Red Clover and Jasmine.

Long/irregular cycles, to help bring on your period and regulate your cycle: Oregano, Basil and Mugwort.

Scanty bleeding: Rosemary, Oregano, Thyme and Motherwort.

Bladder/vaginal infections: Yarrow, Oregano, Lavender, Thyme and Calendula.

Fertility Blend: Rosemary, Basil, Chamomile, Red Rose Petals, Lavender, Calendula, Wormwood and Red Clover.

Blocked fallopian tubes/adhesions: Oregano, Rosemary and Mugwort.

PCOS/ovarian cysts: Rosemary, Motherwort and Lavender.

Endometriosis: Oregano, Motherwort, Yarrow and Rose Petals.

Fibroids: Yarrow, Motherwort, Basil and Calendula.

Pelvic pain: Soothing herbs such as Marshmallow, Calendula and Lavender will relax, soothe and soften the pelvic tissues.

Postpartum: Oregano, Calendula, Motherwort, Rosemary, Red Raspberry Leaf, Basil, Yarrow and Comfrey.

Menopause: Rosemary, Chamomile, Oregano, Raspberry Leaf, Motherwort and Red Rose Petals.

Perineal tear/scars/episiotomy: Calendula, Lavender and Yarrow. Wait until wounds are healed and stitches have been removed.

Miscarriage: Mugwort, Lavender, Calendula, Rosemary, Marigold and Lemon Balm.

Heart and Soul Wise Woman Blend

- 1 tsp Rose Petals
- 1 tsp Mugwort
- 1 tsp Marshmallow Leaf and Roots
- 1 tsp Calendula
- 1 tsp Nettle
- 2 tsp Mint
- 1.5 litres boiling water

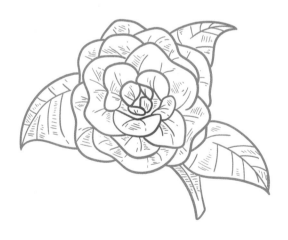

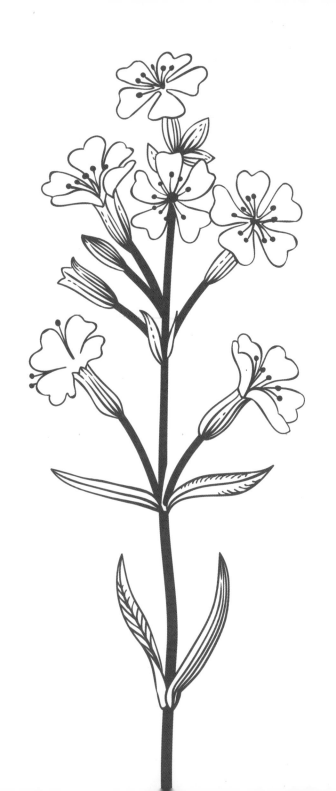

CHAPTER 17

Self-love

When you take the time to honour yourself your womb and your menstrual cycle you may notice the following effects. You may find that your life changes drastically because you no longer suffer from painful menstrual cramps every month. You might develop a greater connection with your body. You might connect with your womb space. Your self-confidence and self-respect might increase.

You may look in the mirror and like who you see. Your eyes may shine. Your stress and worry might fade away. Perhaps the libido you thought had gone forever will return. You could reclaim your sexuality and change the world, your world! You won't know until you try. This is how we will gather the body of evidence to prove that this womb healing medicine works. You are at the forefront of a new wave of women's grassroot medicine that draws from an ancient well of women's wisdom and knowledge of the properties of herbs, water and the love of healing.

෨෨

When you love your womb you reclaim your
energy for self-healing, making yourself whole.
You declare that you are worthy, that you are lovable
and deserving of love.

෨෨

This is a beautiful message to pass onto your children and grandchildren. Ultimately, we must learn to trust our body and our womb's signals and learn to read them before they become symptoms of illness or disease. Imagine a world where young teenagers are introduced to steaming as a self-care ritual to love and honour their bodies; where they are taught about the magic of their menstrual cycle and how to listen to their emerging womb wisdom. This is how healing can pass through generations.

In the future young girls may say, 'I want to be a peri-steam hydrotherapist when I grow up'. Vaginal steaming may become as common as going to the hairdresser or having a pedicure. After all, it is common to spend time on our hair and nails—why not our yonis? Vaginal steams could become part of every hen's party and brides could book in their yoni steams before their big day.

Practitioners will see women in designated clinics and in the privacy of their homes. Postnatal doulas are already offering women yoni steaming as part of their postpartum services. There are V spas where women sit beside each other wrapped up in yoni steam cloaks gossiping over steaming herbs and a cup of tea. This ancient women's wisdom is re-emerging, and what a beautiful time in our evolution for its expansion.

Chapter 18

For Healing and Nurturing

Miscarriage

Your body and your emotions are vulnerable following a miscarriage. At this time the gentle nurturing of a yoni steam will support your body to cleanse and release on a physical and emotional level. Whether a miscarriage is natural or medically assisted, old tissue commonly remains in the uterus. This is known as an incomplete miscarriage. Signs of this condition would include ongoing cramping, missing periods or heavy clotted periods. Steaming will increase blood circulation and encourage the release of any stuck tissue. Wait for bleeding to finish before you do your steam. After your steam, rest, keep warm and give yourself time to process your feelings. Allow healing tears to flow. You may need to forgive your body. Give yourself time. The specific herbs chosen for healing after a miscarriage include Lavender, Rosemary, Marigold and Lemon Balm. The volatile oils of these soothing herbs will help relax the muscles as well as providing nurturing warmth and emotional comfort.

Life after Hysterectomy/Abdominal Surgery

The heating warmth of yoni steaming will help soften and soothe scar tissue and promote healing. When combined with castor oil packs, steaming will increase vitality lost after the operation. Doing a yoni steam at this time helps to energetically and spiritually heal your mind and body after the invasive procedures of surgery. Remember your feminine centre always remains even if you have had your physical womb removed. Your womb's blueprint remains in your energy field. You can no longer conceive a child, though you can still create and birth new ideas, exciting possibilities and grand projects. On an emotional level, give yourself time to reflect and allow yourself to rest before taking on life's busy mantle again.

Post Caesarean or Abdominal Surgery

It is best to wait six weeks or until wounds are healed and stitches have been removed before steaming.

Digestive Issues

Many of us live in a constant state of stress that has a negative impact on digestion. Tension is experienced in the belly as tightness and holding on and is the cause of many digestive ailments such as indigestion, heartburn and constipation. When in 'fight or flight' mode, blood is shunted away from the digestive system and is diverted to the major muscle groups. This decreases the efficiency of food being moved through the body as well as the fluids and secretions that are needed for healthy digestion. Therefore, by taking the time to sit still and relax for ten to twenty minutes while having a yoni steam, you will enjoy the healing benefits of being steamed and soothed by heat and aromatic herbs. You are giving yourself a gift of self-care.

Menstrual Discomfort

Many women experience intense menstrual cramps and discomfort every month when they bleed. They either accept or are told that it is normal. Let me say it again: This is not normal! Steaming has been known to significantly reduce pain bloating and exhaustion associated with your menstrual cycle. Changes to your diet and lifestyle will also help you to recover your physical and emotional equilibrium. Eat wholesome foods and reduce sugar and gluten. Exercise, drink more water and get out in the sun and fresh air. It is recommended to steam two to three times before your period. This will assist your womb to shed its lining. Steam again when you have finished bleeding to help flush everything out.

Premenstrual Tension

Rosita Arvigo tells us that Mayan women drank Rosemary or Basil tea for premenstrual tension. We know that these healing herbs are high in phytoestrogens that are beneficial for PMS. Add them to your yoni steam to ease distressing physical and emotional symptoms.

Scanty Bleeding

Steam during the last week of your cycle before your period with Rosemary, Oregano and Motherwort.

Amenorrhea

When herbs such as Mugwort, Rosemary and Basil are used in combination with the steam, women have reported that their missing period returned after one just steam.

Bacterial Vaginosis

Yoni steaming has been found to be an effective way to treat and prevent PH imbalances including Bacterial Vaginosis, UTI's, yeast infections and excessive bacteria growth. Though scientifically unproven it offers a natural

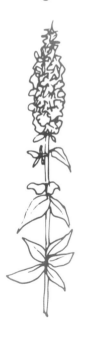

alternative to antibiotics which is the most common way to treat BV. BV is caused by an overgrowth of normal bacteria found in the vagina. Steaming supports the elimination of unhealthy overgrowth bacteria thereby clearing out the excess mucus, the infection and the unpleasant odour that characterises this condition. It also encourages the good flora to reset and prevent future infection. Short steaming sessions of 10 minutes for 10 consecutive days in a row is the recommended regime using astringent herbs that have anti viral, anti bacterial and antimicrobial properties. Lavender, white sage, oregano, mugwort, rose petals, chamomile, mint and calendula may all be used. Please see an Arvigo® practitioner or yoni steam therapist for more guidance.

Female Reproductive Disorders

Ovarian cysts, PCOS and endometriosis may be caused by stagnation of blood lymph and energy flow. Traditional healers and midwives have been treating these female disorders with steaming for centuries.

Fibroids

Uterine fibroids are noncancerous growths of the uterus that often appear during the childbearing years. In Traditional Chinese Medicine, it is believed that stagnation and cold in the pelvic area has a detrimental effect on a woman's health and may contribute to fibroids. Steam combined with herbs helps to soften and warm the tissues to increase energy flow to the womb. Steaming may be done every two weeks but is contraindicated if there is very heavy flooding menses as steaming can increase bleeding.

Pelvic Pain

For women who experience pelvic pain or chronic tension in the pelvic floor, the warmth of steam and herbs will help to soothe and relax the pelvic floor, calm stress hormones and release physical and emotional tension.

Vulvodynia is characterised by burning, pain and discomfort in the vulva with no apparent cause or outward symptoms of infection. For some women with this chronic condition, sex is impossible.

Vaginismus is another distressing condition that causes burning pain and involuntary contractions of the vaginal muscles when sexual intercourse is attempted. In some cases, penetration is intolerable. Causes may be from emotional issues, past abuse or birthing injury. Yoni steams increase circulation to the vulva and will soften and lubricate the vaginal tissues in preparation for lovemaking, allowing sex to be more comfortable and enjoyable. Steaming might also release stored emotions that contribute to these conditions.

Breathing slowly and deeply will calm the nervous system and help to release tension in the jaw as well. The connection between the jaw and the pelvis is now well understood and releasing tension in one will lead to relaxation in the other.

Learning to love and accept yourself as you are will also help you to connect with the sacred energy of your pelvic bowl and your womb space. Your pelvic floor muscles will soften in gratitude and acknowledgement.

Sexual de-armouring: It is now recognised that traumatic life and early childhood experiences can lead to sexual shame and guilt and causes the yoni to become 'armoured'. Armouring is a state of contraction that effectively inhibits the vibrant flow of health, vitality and sexual energy in the pelvic bowl. Due to pain and trauma that has lodged inside the tissues of the body, it has become a survival mechanism to avoid feeling. In doing so, however, the yoni becomes numb and desensitised. The benefits of de-armouring include a renewed lust and joy for life increased sensitivity in the vagina and a deeper connection to one's body and pleasure zones. Hand in hand with the emerging modalities of yoni massage and yoni mapping, steaming is a gift to women to help them come back into their bodies and reclaim their sexuality and sensuality.

CHAPTER 19

Yoni Steaming for Fertility

Many women struggle to conceive and endure months and years of disappointment and heartache. One of the factors that may possibly have been overlooked is poor circulation or lack of blood flow to the womb. Our sedentary lifestyles contribute to this along with poor diet being overweight or underweight and stressed. The endometrium needs good blood flow to be plump and nourished to receive and implant an embryo. Steams may be particularly helpful when women have dark or brown blood at the beginning or the end of their cycle. This is a sign that the womb has not emptied out completely from the last cycle. The plant oils and the steam encourage the body to slough off old blood and tissue that rests in the hills and valleys of the uterine wall enabling the womb to grow a fresh healthy lining during the next cycle.

Vaginal Steaming brings heat to the womb and this practice is becoming increasingly popular among women trying to conceive as a means of enhancing circulation, relieving congestion and detoxifying the womb.

Steaming is an integral modality of the Arvigo Techniques of Maya Abdominal Therapy® and many women have successfully conceived when they make lifestyle changes and take steps to cleanse their wombs. In the USA, where this practice is more well known, fertility clinics offer steams as a complementary therapy for women undergoing in-vitro fertilisation or intra-uterine insemination. The doctors are asking for this as they have found it is easier to insert their instruments if steaming is done prior to the procedures.

⤶

There may be many reasons for infertility, but one of those reasons is induration of the uterine wall. When we combine vaginal steaming with abdominal therapy – the deep external massage on the uterus – we have a very dynamic approach with great results.

—Rosita Arvigo, DN

⤶

Unblock Fallopian Tubes

Blockages of the fallopian tubes can be a contributing cause of infertility. The fallopian tubes are thin tubules lined with cilia—tiny hairs that help the egg travel down from the ovary to the womb in one direction and waft the sperm up towards the egg in the other direction. As most fertilisation occurs here, it is vital the tubes remain healthy and clear. Surgery, endometriosis, previous infection and sexually transmitted disease can all cause scar tissue that block the tubes. A build-up of old blood and residue in the uterus may also obstruct the entrance. Steaming with antibacterial herbs combined with abdominal massage to increase circulation will reduce inflammation and help break up scar tissue.

Increase Fertile Cervical Fluid

Long-term use of the hormonal birth control pill can dry a woman's crypts (the cells in the cervix that produce cervical fluid) making things 'less juicy' down there. Adequate cervical fluid is needed to speed sperm on its way through the uterus to the fallopian tubes in order for conception to occur. Women have noticed a significant increase in cervical fluids after steaming. The steam will also thin excess mucus, leaving behind only vital, fertile fluids.

Sweeten Your Yoni Nectar

It may be harder to become pregnant when diet and lifestyle have created an acidic environment in the body. An acidic environment inside the vagina may mean that the cervical mucus is killing off the sperm. Yoni steaming will help balance the delicate vaginal ecosystem. Due to the natural detoxifying effects of the steam your yoni secretions will naturally begin to taste and smell sweeter as your body moves towards a more alkaline state.

Stress Relief

Yoni steaming provides support and nurturing warmth when life is fraught with stress and anxiety. It is a self-care practice that you can do in the privacy of your own home where nobody is telling you what is wrong with you or what procedure or test to do next. The soothing fragrant steam activates your parasympathetic nervous system, calms your nerves and softens the internal membranes so that they are moist and receptive to conception.

A Fertility Blend to encourage cervical mucus production:

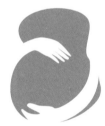

- ½ tsp Red Clover
- 1 tsp Dandelion Leaf
- ½ tsp Motherwort
- 1 tsp Red Raspberry Leaf
- 1.5 litres water

Best Time to Steam for Fertility Enhancement

The ideal time to steam to prepare for conception is before ovulation. This will make sure the tissues are moist and the cervical fluids are clear and copious. Do not steam after ovulation or when there is any possibility that you might be pregnant. You can steam for three days in a row at the beginning of your cycle once you have finished bleeding. You may repeat in the last week of your cycle, but only if you are not trying to conceive in that cycle.

Again, steaming is contraindicated during the second half of the cycle if there is any possibility of pregnancy.

How the Arvigo® Techniques can Further Enhance Fertility

We have seen how Arvigo® massage moves congested lymph fluid, boosts immune function and increases blood circulation to the pelvic organs. Regardless of the complaints that a woman or couple presents with on their fertility journey, when they receive an Arvigo® session, the intention will always be to encourage the five flows to the abdominal area, especially the uterus, the ovaries, the fallopian tubes. The optimum flows of arterial, venous, nerve, lymphatic and *chulel,* the Maya word for chi, will help cleanse, prepare and build a healthy uterine lining. As Rosita says, this is like preparing the crib with loving intentions for your baby.

'One of the Arvigo® protocols for fertility enhancement is a three-month program that combines professional treatments, yoni steams and self-care massage. During this time, while the body is being given every chance to renew, cleanse and regenerate, couples are actively encouraged *not* to conceive.

'There is also a one-month protocol for couples who do not wish to stop trying to conceive. This includes the massage sessions, yoni steams and self-care in the first half of the cycle between menstruation and ovulation. Whether you commit to the one-month or the three-month program the goal is the same: uterine lavage to cleanse the uterine membrane and realignment of the reproductive organs to their optimal positions. Arvigo® therapy is a gentle non-invasive modality that will support and optimise your chances of conception.

To find out more and hopefully find an Arvigo® practitioner near you go to www.arvigotherapy.com

୭୧

*Give nature half a chance, and there
is a miracle in store for everyone.*

— Rosita Arvigo, DN

୭୧

Spring Cleaning

Having a yoni steam is essentially decluttering your womb. Just like when you declutter your house, steaming every month is an opportunity to let go of the past, enjoy the present, and clear the way for new energy to come in.

We have already considered that your menstrual cycle is a reflection of your overall health. On the physical level, every month your womb releases the lining that is no longer needed if conception does not occur. On an emotional level, you have the opportunity to do the same. In your mind you can consciously release the thought forms, events and actions of the past few weeks. What did you achieve? What didn't work for you? Did you honour your boundaries? Did you stand up for yourself? Were your thoughts about yourself (and others) positive? How was your relationship with food, sex and money? This is not a time to beat yourself up. No judgements!

This helps to prepare for the new month ahead. What would you like to create and achieve? This might be a new business, relationship or creative endeavour. This is the opportunity your menstrual cycle offers you every month.

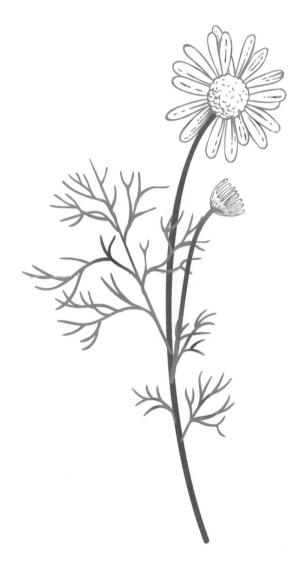

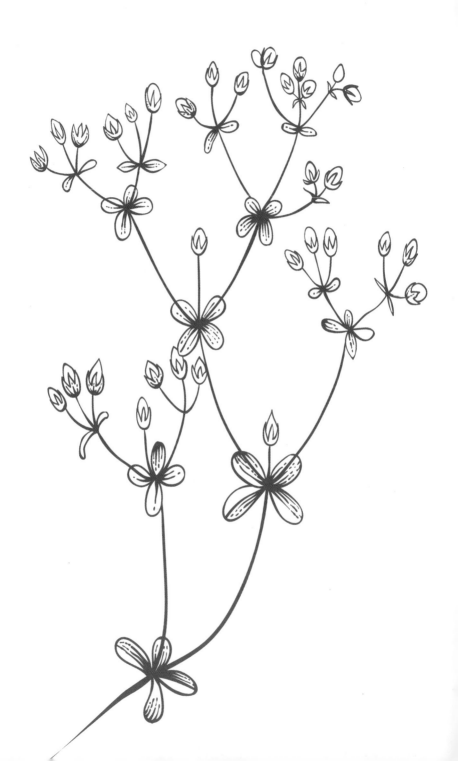

Chapter 20

Healing Past Trauma with Yoni Steaming

EMOTIONAL ISSUES

Many women are disconnected from their bodies due to past trauma and abuse. This may mean that they feel cut off from the lower part of their body in order to unconsciously protect themselves from past trauma. A woman's womb holds onto old hurts, disappointment and heartbreak. Unhappy experiences, abortion, rape, rejection and unwanted memories of past partners are all stored in the tissues. This gentle method of self-care helps heal the spirit as well as the body.

When used with ceremony and a spirit of honouring the beautiful herbs and the blessed water, the efficacy is even more powerful. The gentle energy of steam and herbs combined will help to soothe, recover and renew from trauma and abuse. Sometimes there may be an emotional reaction after your steam, as the armouring and tension that has long been stored to protect you is released. Allow the tears to flow. Seek loving support at this time. Be gentle with yourself.

Sexual Abuse

Too many women have experienced trauma through sexual abuse, incest and rape. This has a lasting effect throughout her life by disturbing and disrupting her natural healthy energy flow. As more women find the courage to speak up about their trauma (sometimes decades later) we are finding new holistic ways to help survivors. We live in an age where quantum physics back up what healers have always intrinsically known. It is now recognised that trauma gets lodged in our DNA and in our tissues and if not addressed may show up as disease.

ᘒ

Your issues are in your tissues.

ᘒ

Quantum healing states it is possible to create a healing environment for ourselves that will literally change the energetic make up of our cells. WOW! We can also change the mindset that is necessary to facilitate ongoing healing. This is way beyond the scope of this book about herbs and steam, but the practice of yoni steaming is surely a tool in your medicine bag to help your restorative journey. It is but one way that we can take responsibility for our health, include energy medicine and holistic methods of health care into our lives.

There are practitioners who specifically offer guided vaginal steam sessions to help sexual abuse survivors. This is done in a safe space with the consent of the woman and with the intention to heal and release sexual trauma. When somebody has experienced sexual abuse, their body continues to operate in chronic, low-grade 'fight or flight' mode. There is an interplay between the parasympathetic nervous system, the psoas muscle, the vagus nerve and the abdominal viscera including the reproductive organs.

Vaginal steaming relaxes the viscera and the nervous system, which help a woman's recovery and health. The vagus nerve conducts sensory information directly from the cervix to the brain. Since the steam rises and eventually reaches the cervix, it makes sense that the vagus nerve is stimulated. This in turn will releases high levels of oxytocin known as the 'trust hormone' or the 'love hormone' which directly sends neurotransmissions to the brain to make somebody happy and get the body out of 'fight, flight or freeze'. This is backed up by scientific research (see Resources).

Women have begun to use yoni steaming to cleanse themselves of unwanted memories of past partners, sexual abuse and rape. However, this book does not claim that yoni steaming alone will be able to undo the long-term physical and emotional damage caused by sexual abuse. The negative effects on mind, body and spirit are far reaching and for many it is a long road to recovery that requires ongoing trauma resolution and professional advocacy. Please seek professional help if a yoni steam triggers memories of abuse.

A Womb Never Forgets

Your womb has been with you through your whole life. She was within you as a baby with all your eggs intact, and with you at your menarche, your first sexual experience, throughout your relationships, the births of your children, literally in sickness and in health. She knows you better than anyone. She is you. She has been with you through the good and the bad. She remembers you falling in love and having great sex. She remembers you feeling lonely and insecure. She may have also witnessed abuse, disappointment, fertility challenges, miscarriages, abortions and sexually transmitted diseases. She has felt your anger, resentment, sadness, shame, self-loathing and lack of forgiveness towards others and yourself. Your heart is intimately connected with your womb.

According to Chinese Medicine, there is a direct channel called the 'uterus vessel' or the *bao mai* that connects the two. There is a saying that when your heart breaks, your womb breaks. This is why. Your womb remembers it all. Until you are able to acknowledge heartache and let go of emotional and mental triggers every month, she may cry out in pain in the symptoms of menstrual cramps, reproductive ailments and fertility challenges. She will struggle with the load.

୬ଙ୬

Energetically, your emotions are stored in your heart and your womb. The womb, for a woman, is her second heart.

When women don't have the tools to deal with their emotions, the womb stores what we haven't processed.

୬ଙ୬

An Attitude of Forgiveness

The act of forgiveness allows you to release toxic emotions in order to clear your energetic womb space much like the steam and herbs clear the physical womb. When you cleanse your womb space it allows you to be free to create what you want for yourself and your life: just like the Feng Shui principle of clearing away your clutter to make room for the new.

The next time you steam, close your eyes and say to yourself:

- *I forgive those who have hurt me knowingly or unknowingly.*

- *I forgive myself for hurting others knowingly or unknowingly.*

- *I forgive myself for hurting myself.*

Imagine toxins and emotional trauma being removed from your yoni. If anybody appears in your mind's eye, view them like an actor on the stage and declare your willingness to forgive them (even if you doubt your ability to do so). Even if you are angry with someone, imagine seeing them surrounded with the pink light of forgiveness and encourage them to disappear. Eliminate them from your body, mind and auric field once and for all. You may find this really challenging and you may not want to do this. There is no judgement here. It may not happen in one steam. It may take three, four, six or ten steams combined with other healing modalities to assist you. Ask for help in letting go. Forgiveness is not about condoning a person's actions—ever. It is a healing process that will set you free. Acknowledge emotions that may arise and tears that may flow.

Tapping for forgiveness

The Emotional Freedom Technique (EFT), also known as tapping, is a tool that can be used to help you reduce stress and promote a positive outlook. It is described as 'psychological acupuncture without the needles'. The beauty of this method is that it is literally at your fingertips, which you can use any time, any place, anywhere. Tapping utilises the body's energy meridian points by stimulating them with your fingertips—literally tapping into your body's own energy and healing power. Tapping, steaming and practicing forgiveness is a powerful combination.

For more information on tapping see Resources.

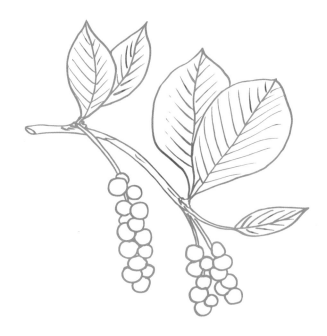

CHAPTER 21

Body Image

It is a sad fact that many women do not love their bodies. And even sadder that women like their genitalia even less and find it hard to talk about their vagina and their periods. Many women feel insecure about how their vulva looks and smells. There is a huge range of feminine hygiene products available to cleanse, douche and powder your genitals in order to mask their natural smell.

Women of all ages aspire to have the glossy hair, flawless skin, legs, hips and breasts of the models seen in the media. A common misconception is the expectation for perfection, including a perfect vulva. Women are signing up for cosmetic surgery 'down there' in droves because they do not like the size or shape of their vulvas. Designer vaginas have become the new trend and some women spend thousands of dollars on risky, painful, plastic surgery to make their unique genitalia look more like the unrealistic vulvas portrayed in porn movies.

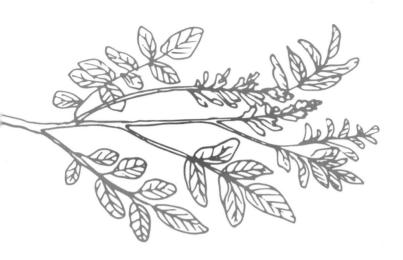

Vaginal steaming is not the answer to everything. By itself it may not cure women's shame and low self-esteem. It is a time-honoured traditional therapy that has been used in cultures all over the world in every phase of a woman's life. It is a practice that women have always shared together in the privacy of the home or the hut in the village. Mothers passed on this wisdom to their daughters and they in turn imparted the knowledge to their daughters.

My fervent wish is that it becomes a tool for every woman to add to her medicine bag to aid and empower her to love and feel at home in her body and at peace with her menstrual flow every month. Yoni steaming can be part of a healthy lifestyle that includes exercising, eating well and balancing work and play.

꧁꧂

*When you connect with prayer and intention
to the plants, the water and the steam, you connect
to the healing energy of Mother Earth.*

꧁꧂

Whether you believe in the magic or not, making the connection to your own womb and to the earth will have a profound influence in your life and in the lives of generations to come.

༄

When you heal yourself, you heal your ancestral and future generations.

༄

Every woman needs to be told about this natural solution to her reproductive health challenges. It is time to take your own health into your hands to lay your own hands on your womb and find gentle non-harmful methods to heal your reproductive ailments. I encourage you to try it for yourself, if not for yourself then for your future children or grandchildren.

༄

Your womb is so much more than the place in which physical life is created, nurtured and brought forth into the world. Not only is human life conceived and grown within the womb, but your innermost dreams and desires are conceived here too.

༄

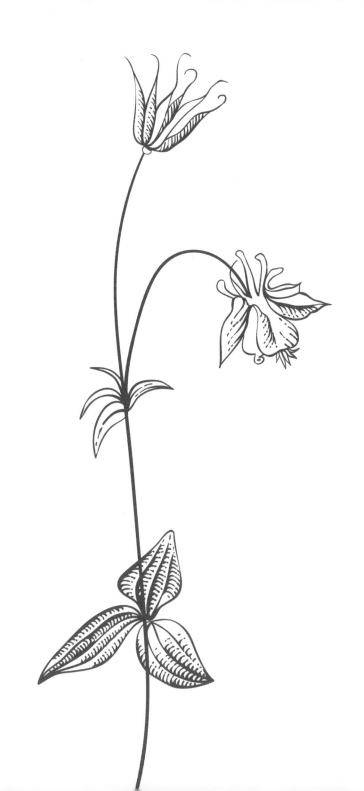

CHAPTER 22

Womb Affirmations

Louise Hay taught us that our lives reflect the beliefs we hold. Louise was a modern pioneer in teaching us that we can change our lives through affirmations. Affirmations can be a useful tool in helping change beliefs. When you replace old, outmoded beliefs about yourself with new, positive intentions, you will discover a new healing ally inside your mind and womb. When these new positive thoughts take root, and become habits, the shift that will occur can be profound and life changing ... for the better.

- I am a strong and capable woman.
- I am safe.
- I am grounded.

- I am comfortable, calm and in control.
- I accept myself completely here and now.
- I love and accept my body completely.
- I am grateful for the blessings in my life.
- I love my womb.
- All is well with my world.

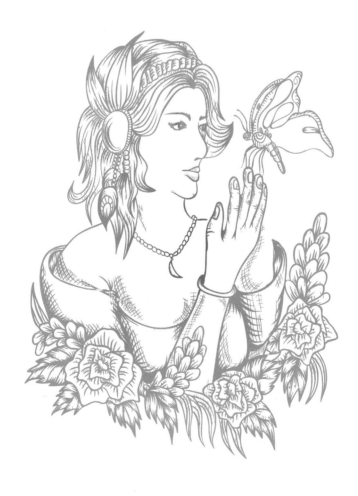

Womb Medicine

Chapter 23

More About the Arvigo Techniques of Maya Abdominal Therapy®

The Arvigo Techniques of Maya Abdominal Therapy® and Spiritual Healing are inspired by traditional Maya healing techniques. These techniques were developed over time by Dr Rosita Arvigo based on her apprenticeship with the Maya Healer and Shaman Don Elijio Panti, her own deep love of plant medicine and her training as a naprapathic physician. She combined her knowledge of anatomy, physiology, herbs, and napropathy with the traditional methods of her teachers to adapt this healing modality for modern times. Rosita has devoted her whole life to the study of healing and plant medicine and is the author of many wonderful books on herb lore. Her latest book, the Urban Herbalist, is a guide to medicinal herbs found in industrialised cities both in America and Australia.

Benefits for Your Womb

Arvigo® abdominal massage is an external, gentle series of moves that help to reposition internal organs of the digestive and reproductive system. It is best known for helping to shift the uterus back into optimal balance in the pelvic bowl.

Repositioning organs that have moved out of alignment helps to restore healthy and optimal blood, lymph, nerve and energy flow within the body. This massage helps to support the body's natural healing capacity when things are out of balance and to prevent dis-ease within the body before it happens.

Old adhesions and scar tissue from invasive treatments to the pelvis will soften and dissolve. This will help reproductive ailments that many women have been suffering from for years. These may include fibroid tumours, endometriosis, digestive, urinary and bladder problems. In addition to physically releasing deep tension and refreshing the blood flow to muscles and organs, abdominal massage reopens blocked energy paths and releases blocked chi that has accumulated due to pent-up emotions.

The blood vessels of the womb are beautifully interwoven and lie close to the uterus and ovaries. Only five per cent of blood goes to the womb and the Arvigo® massage is an effective way to increase circulation.

Mind Your Own Womb

Take some time today to listen to your womb and appreciate her. The abdomen is an area where many women store negative repressed emotions such as anxiety, fear, shame, resentment, grief, and anger. When these emotions are constantly suppressed, muscular armouring occurs which shuts down emotional expression even more. The body responds to fear over a lifetime by shutting down and going into survival mode.

Tami Lynn Kent, author of *Wild Feminine* suggests that pelvic health is connected to the base chakra (the chakra that sits in the pelvic bowl and governs feelings of security and belonging) and has a bearing on a woman's wellbeing. When a woman feels safe, her pelvic floor muscles (same as her other muscles) are relaxed; when afraid or tense, they tighten. Constriction in this area will affect a woman's connection to her sexuality, creativity and life itself, often on an unconscious level.

Keep Calm and Rub Your Belly

In Western culture we are not taught how to properly take care of our bodies, particularly our wombs, to prevent disease. It is probably not such a farfetched statement to say that we know how to service our cars better than we know how to take care of our uterine health. What if we had the tools to maintain our bodies?

When you receive a session of the Arvigo Techniques of Maya Abdominal Therapy®, you will be taught how to do self-care massage at home. Self-care massage is one of the easiest and cheapest ways to improve uterine health, break-up and prevent adhesions and scar tissue and promote healing of the uterus. By practicing abdominal self-care massage, you can prevent future disease from occurring, much like brushing your teeth helps to maintain dental health. It can be done in the comfort and privacy of your own home either the first thing in the morning or before you go to sleep (or whenever you choose!). When you have had your womb guided back to her optimal position through yoni steaming, following it up with self-care massage will help maintain the muscles and ligaments in a healthy position. If you don't, the muscles will naturally move back into the incorrect position again after years of being that way. This is an extraordinary self-help tool that can be used to support and promote your personal womb health and wellbeing. It is a gift you give yourself.

ᘓᕒᕒ

Nourish your womb into vibrant health!

ᘓᕒᕒ

Self-care Massage

Self-care massage is an opportunity to honour yourself and your body. Gifting yourself this precious time, bestowing love and appreciation for your body, and paying attention to what she may be wishing to communicate with you, is an act of self-love that imbues feelings of calmness and kindness. Through regular practice of yoni steaming and self-care massage you will notice a reduction in mind chatter which may be feeding your inner critic by playing endless loops of 'not good enough, pretty enough, skinny enough' etc. Utilise this time to affirm the beauty of your womanhood and all that you are grateful for, including the precious water and healing herbs you may be using in your steam. Use gentle, slow, soft stroking motions during your self-care massage, and most importantly ensure it feels pleasurable!

Testimonials

The following testimonial is from Kate, a thirty-year-old Australian woman who works on a remote aboriginal community in Central Australia. In 2017 she had a routine pap smear that revealed low-grade changes that were diagnosed as cervical dysplasia, also referred to as precancer. A subsequent biopsy revealed a lesion caused by the HPV virus and surgery was recommended. After doing extensive research into natural healing modalities, she decided to embark on a yoni steaming routine and chose Calendula, White Peony Root, Sage, Rosemary, Corn Silk, Lemon Balm, Yarrow and Holy Basil as her therapeutic herbs. She steamed in fifteen to twenty-minute increments every day for two weeks, and then three times a week following that. When she returned to the hospital two months later to assess her situation, the lesion had completely disappeared.

'Yoni steaming has helped me immensely! Since steaming my whole cycle and blood quality has changed. My blood is so much healthier and vibrant! Steaming is a place I connect to my

internal space to connect to the Divine inside and out. I love working with herbs and prayer in this ritual. Now I steam nearly every fortnight and it has become part of my health and hygiene practice. Like getting a massage or brushing my teeth! I do believe it is a missing link in our complete self-care.'

Melissa a massage therapist who steams every month as part of her self-care regime says:

'I love the whole sensuality of yoni steaming. I feel it connects me to my essential female nature. I can feel the warmth and the energy spiralling upwards and afterwards I feel deeply relaxed and expansive.'

Sam, an acupuncturist, says:

'I didn't know what to think about this vaginal steaming business. I was quite sceptical until I tried it! Oh my, things felt ten years younger down there after just one steam and this pleasant feeling lasted for two weeks!'

Resources

Purchasing Yoni Steam Herbs

Many health food shops stock herbs in bulk and sell organic herbs like Oregano, Basil, Calendula, Lavender, Red Raspberry Leaf, etc.

Shakti Whispers Herb Blends

Tracy Whitton is the founder of Stillness Through Movement and the Feminine Embodiment Technique that blends esoteric breast and womb massage with yoni steaming. https://www.stmt.com.au

Heart and Soul Herbs

Special herb blends grown in our garden in Nobby's Creek and blended specifically for yoni steaming are available for sale. Blends are available for different needs. www.heartandsoulofwellness.com.au

Guided Womb Meditations

www.spaceinbetween.com.au
www.soulvibrance.com
www.thesacredwomb.com

You can purchase and download the above meditations online. YouTube is also a great resource, providing infinite hours of free stuff to listen to. Tune in to which ones you resonate with.

Tapping

For information on Tapping visit:
www.thetappingsolution.com

Further Information

For information on Arvigo® courses and workshops in Australia contact the Arvigo Institute on:
www.arvigotherapy.com

Many Arvigo® Practitioners offer yoni steams as part of their therapy sessions. More information about the Arvigo Techniques of Maya Abdominal Therapy® and Arvigo® practitioners can be found on the following websites:
www.arvigotherapy.com
www.heartandsoulofwellness.com.au

Additional Resources

Gaza, Keli: Steamy Chick,
www.steamychick.com

Spink, Clare: Womb & Fertility Massage
www.fertilitymassage.co.uk

References

Memeh, Ijeoma Sophia *Healing through Vaginal Steaming*, USA, 2011

Arvigo, Rosita and Epstein, Nadine, *Rainforest Home Remedies: The Maya Way to Heal your Body and Replenish Your Soul*, Harper Collins, San Francisco, 2001

Arvigo, Rosita and Epstein,Nadine, *Spiritual Bathing*, Vermont, Echo Points and Media, 2018

Arvigo Rosita, *The Urban Herbalist: A Guide to Medicinal Plants*, Story Bridge Books, 2018

Kent, Tami Lynn, *Wild Feminine*, New York, Simon & Schuster Inc, 2011

Harris, Karen and Caskey-Sigety, Lori: *The Medieval Vagina: A Hysterical and Historical Perspective of all Things Vaginal During the Middle Ages*, Indiana, Snark Publishing, Indiana USA, 2014

Green, Monica. H. *The Trotula*, Philadelphia, University of Pennsylvania Press, 2002

Isaacs Jennifer, *Bush Food, Aboriginal Food and Herbal Medicine*, Sydney, Australia, Landsdowne Publishing Pty. Ltd, 1996

Whitton, Tracy, *Feminine Embodiment Level 1 Therapy, Guidelines for a feminine-focused practice for all ages and stages of a woman's life cycle*, Stillness Through Movement, Gold Coast, Queensland, Australia, 2019

Arvigo, Rosita You Tube: Vaginal Steams for Preconception and Postpartum with Rosita Arvigo, http://www.birth-institute.com

Vagal afferents from the uterus and cervix provide direct connections to the brainstem https://www.ncbi.nlm.nih.gov/pubmed/9931352

Ix Chel

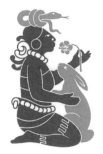

The resurgence of feminine consciousness was predicted by the Maya to begin in 2012. Before the revival of these teachings, Ix Chel was largely an unnoticed goddess of the Americas, hidden in the mists of time. Thanks to Rosita Arvigo, she is no longer a forgotten Goddess and Ix Chel, the Goddess of Medicine and the Moon, has become the patroness of the Arvigo® lineage. Her image is portrayed as one aspect of the triple goddess, either Maiden, Mother or Crone.

About the Author

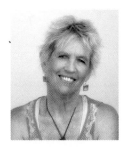

Sali is a certified Arvigo® Practitioner and Educator and creatrix of the Heart and Soul of Wellness Centre in Murwillumbah, NSW, Australia. She is grandmother, mother, partner, sister, friend, aunty and wise woman. A perpetual student of life, she is endlessly fascinated by these human bodies we inhabit, our energetic and spiritual make up and metaphysical anatomy. She is inspired by babies, little children, Mother Earth, Women's Wisdom and Old Wives Tales. She loves herbs, crystals, angels, trees, dragons and faeries. She is a pre natal yoga teacher, midwife, childbirth educator and birth physiology nerd. Having birthed four babies at home in the eighties, she is passionate about educating and preparing women for labour, birth and for becoming new mamas. She offers free postpartum yoni steaming for women in the postnatal Mums n' Bubs group in Murwillumbah.

She lives with her partner Gerry and their staffy Mac in Nobby's Creek in Northern NSW where they manage a retreat space for yoga and wellness retreats. She feels privileged to be caretaker of this beautiful land and loves to walk the tracks in the forest. Above all she loves to grow herbs and create new gardens. She is awed and amazed by the practical wisdom and healing that ancient techniques offer and is equally inspired by the new modalities of healing and energy medicine that are evolving.

To find out more about Sali, go to
www.heartandsoulofwellness.com.au

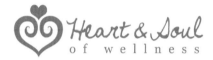

Coming titles by the author

Womb Medicine Healing Cards – 2020

Your Uterus Knows Best – 2021

About the Cover Artist

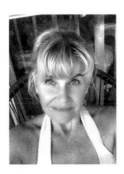

Melissa is a trained graphic designer and worked as an art director in her life before children. Artistic expression is her natural talent and it is her great love to create art, simply for the joy of what comes through. It is a wonderful gift to bring ideas, feelings and experiences into form on an empty page.

Melissa is contactable for commissions via email
Melissa.juchau@gmail.com

Notes